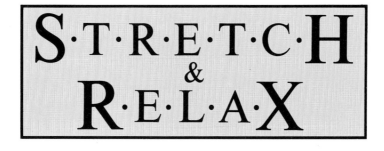

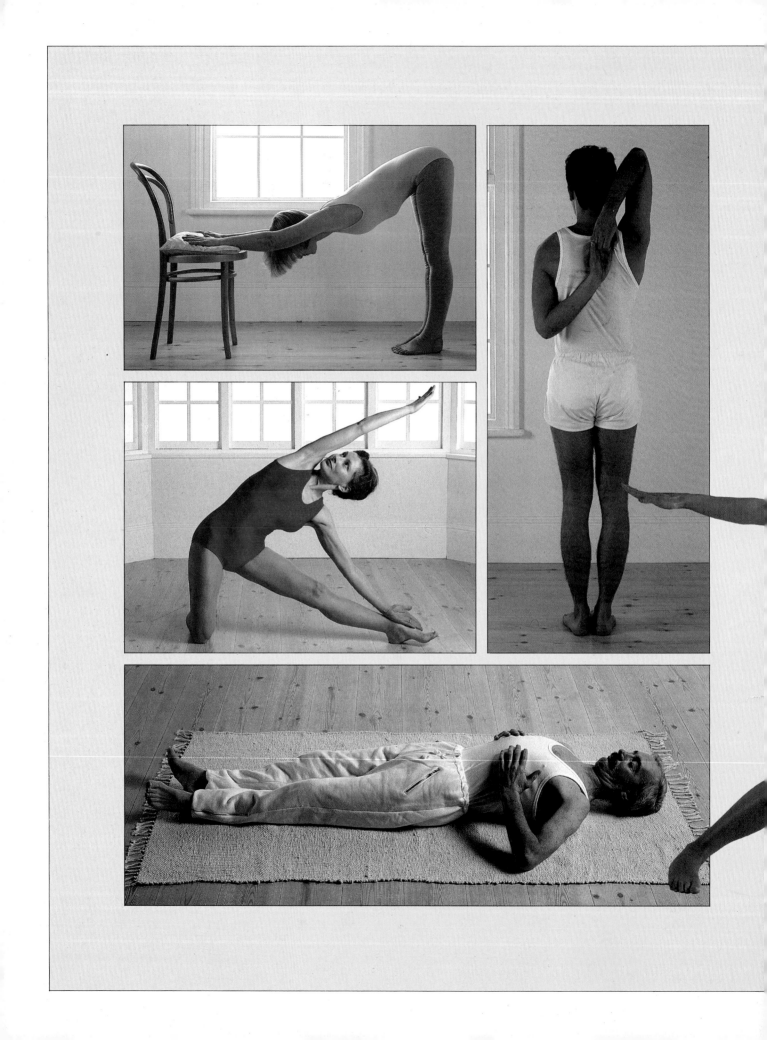

S·T·R·E·T·C·H
&
R·E·L·A·X

·MAXINE TOBIAS· & ·MARY STEWART·

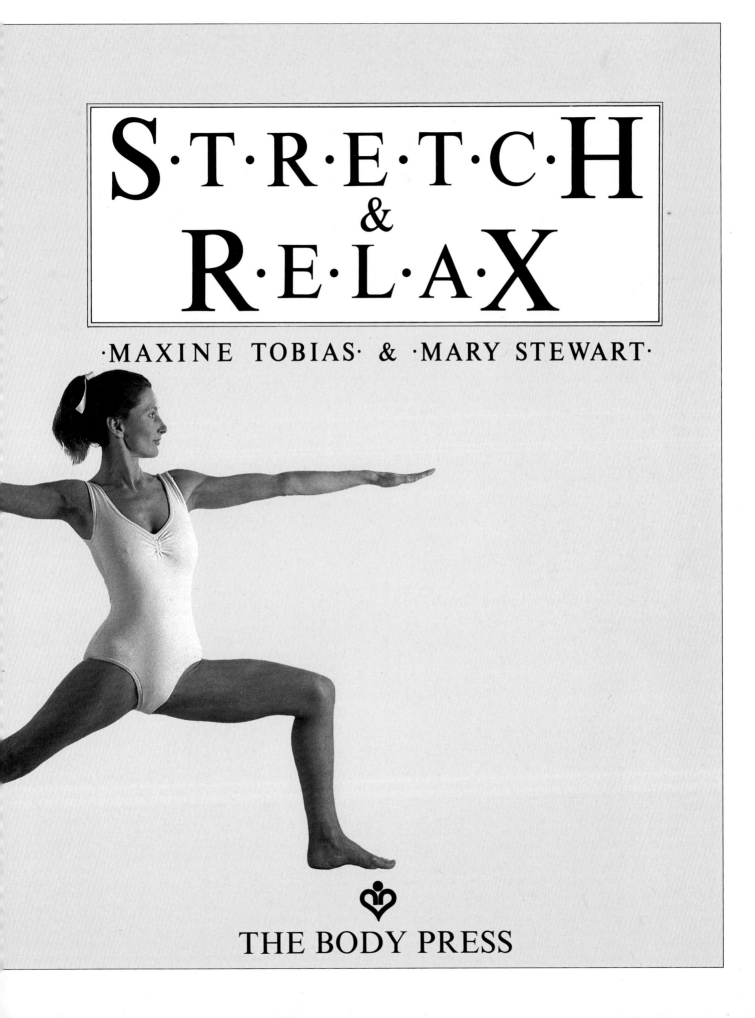

THE BODY PRESS

First published in Great Britain in 1985 by
Dorling Kindersley Publishers Limited,
9 Henrietta Street, London WC2E 8PS

Publisher: Rick Bailey
Editorial Director: Randy Summerlin
Editor: Judith Schuler
Technical Consultant: Mary Anne Newell, M.S., M.Ed.

The Body Press, a division of HPBooks, Inc.
P.O. Box 5367
Tucson, AZ 85703
(602) 888-2150

ISBN: 0-89586-416-9

Library of Congress Catalog Card Number: 85-60489
1st Printing

Typeset by Chambers Wallace, London.
Printed in Italy by Arnoldo Mondadori, Verona.

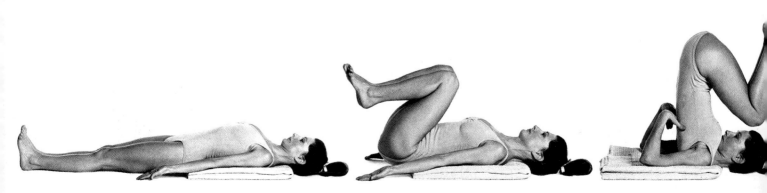

·CONTENTS·

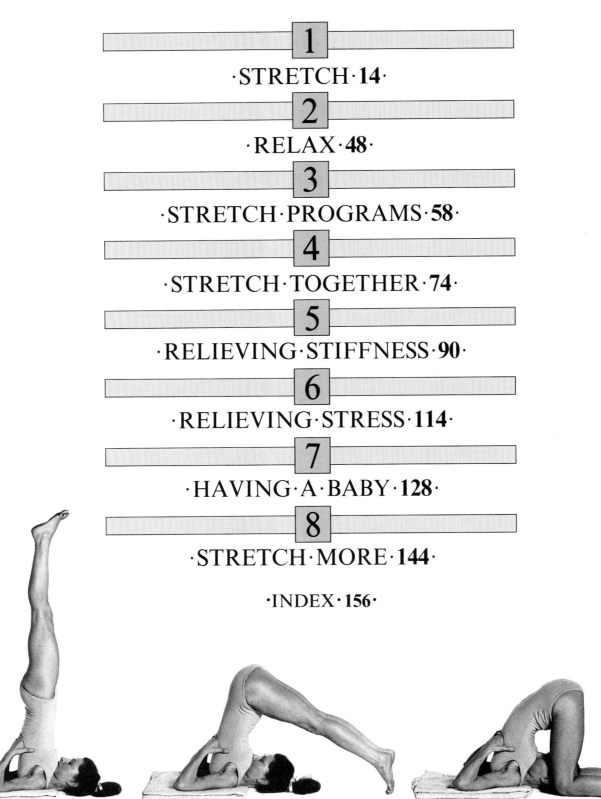

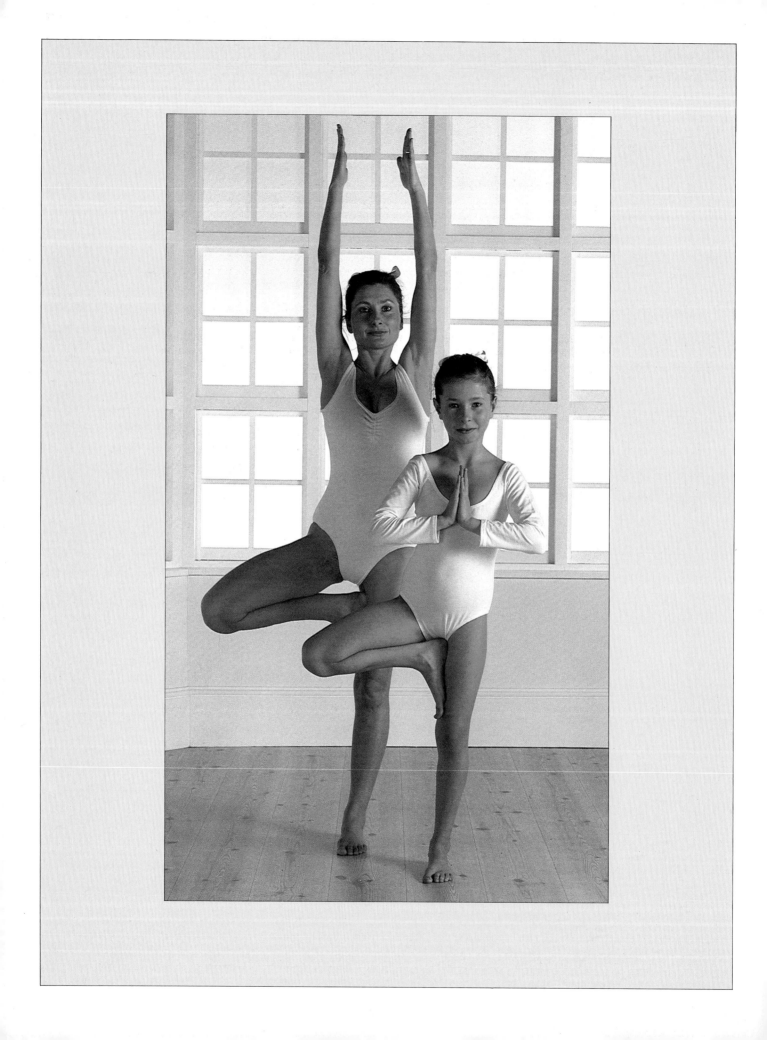

· ABOUT · THE · AUTHORS ·

· MARY · STEWART ·

I started practicing yoga in the mid-60s from a book. The small amount of practice I did each day revolutionized my life. This is one reason I wanted to write a book; there must be thousands of people like me who would never have gone to a class in the beginning. I began attending classes in 1968.

In 1969, I attended a teachers' training course and Maxine and I met in the class. We were studying the Iyengar method, and B.K.S. Iyengar came from India for one month, once a year, to supervise the training program.

When I first began teaching, I taught in various adult education institutes. After a few years I started teaching privately, hiring church halls for classes. This allowed me to teach smaller groups and to grade students in my classes. I also taught yoga in a London teaching hospital and in two other establishments.

Maxine and I studied with Dona Holleman in Italy. To give others the benefit of what we learned, we started a teachers' training class in London. This was for those preparing to take the Iyengar teaching certificate and also for those already teaching who wanted to advance. Today, pupils from these classes are teaching all over the world.

My personality is different from Maxine's. We have held many courses and workshops together, mostly for teachers. Students seem to benefit from our two different approaches. I have also given courses in Italy and in France, and last year I taught in South Africa when I was in Cape Town visiting my daughter.

I became interested in teaching yoga to pregnant women when a pupil of mine and I arranged for Dr. Leboyer from Paris to give a lecture on birth for yoga teachers. I later helped produce a poster of yoga positions for pregnancy.

· MAXINE · TOBIAS ·

After studying yoga in Paris on my own from books, I took classes in London from a teacher who had been a pupil of B.K.S. Iyengar. My first meeting with Mr Iyengar himself and the classes I took with him really fired my imagination and enthusiasm. His precision and dynamic energy were the key to his teaching, and I became an ardent student. I studied with him in London and Poona (India) where he now has a Yoga Institute.

I met Mary Stewart at the teachers' training classes. After working with Dona Holleman, a senior Iyengar teacher in Italy, Mary and I started training teachers together in the 70s. We both served on the committee for the B.K.S. Iyengar Teachers' Association, and I edited their newsletter. I have also trained and assessed trainee teachers.

Mary and I found that our methods of working complemented each other, which is a rare phenomenon. Together, we have held workshops and trained teachers at elementary and intermediate levels. We are both rooted in the traditions of our own culture and religion and are not interested in quasi-mysticism or the "Eastern way of Life." This prompted us to write this book. Even though we are committed to our own practice, not everyone wants to follow the path of yoga but would benefit enormously from its practice.

As an aid to training teachers, we have studied the "Ramayana" at the Bharatiya Vidya Bhavan, studied and taught "The Yoga Sutras of Patanjali" to our trainee teachers and read other material relating to the subject of yoga and Indian studies.

·INTRODUCTION·

Stretch and Relax is based on yoga, which we both practice and teach. Yoga has never been primarily a method of keeping fit, although health and mental stability are the results of yoga that is practiced correctly. Because this book is based on the ancient system, it isn't intended to make you conform to a particular standard of physical fitness or fashionable look. Instead, you should find yourself at ease with your body as you strengthen muscles and improve posture. Practiced regularly, the *Stretch and Relax* system promotes good health, whatever your physical type. It increases your stamina, reduces fatigue and makes you more resistant to stress and minor physical ailments.

·ENJOY·STRETCHING·EVERY·DAY·

You may be inspired to start a fitness program by some fantasy image of how you would like to look or behave. Reality soon catches up with you, and you give up, disheartened and disillusioned. Or you may hurt your body by forcing it to conform to an unrealistic ideal. This book is based on the practical needs of men and women in everyday life. The stretches, relaxation and breathing techniques can be started by anyone, at any time in life. This is not a rigid discipline designed to punish your body; it's an enjoyable way of releasing tensions and improving your health through an evolving method you tailor to suit your individual needs.

The people who come to our regular classes are from all walks of life and perform many kinds of jobs. The main thing they have in common is they lead busy lives without much time for themselves. Working with them over the years, we have seen those who practice regularly, even if for a few minutes a day, derive more benefit than those who only attend a class for a weekly workout. Regular practice is the basis of *Stretch and Relax*.

·ANYONE·CAN·STRETCH·

But practicing regularly is not always easy. You need to be motivated by a positive attitude toward your body and its use. Many students have asked us for a daily program to help them start practicing when they don't feel like it. As a result, we have devised this system of graded stretches, designed to be an enjoyable way of taking your body through the full range of physical movements. The system can be followed by anyone, from stiff beginners to gymnasts. As long as you practice regularly and sensibly, you can adapt the system as your flexibility improves. Your practice progresses and does not become dull or stale.

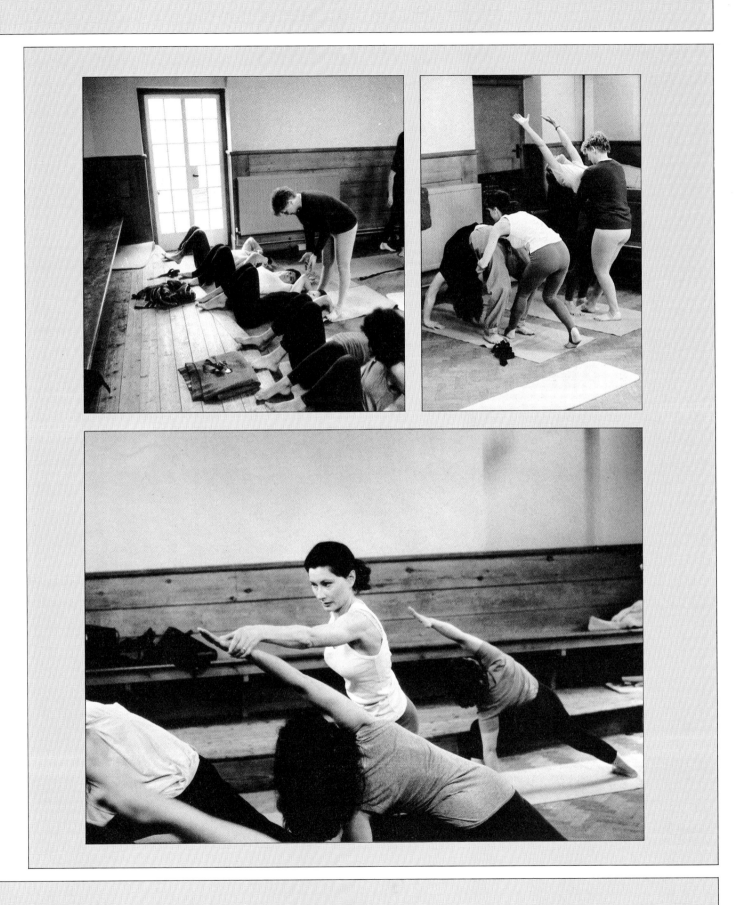

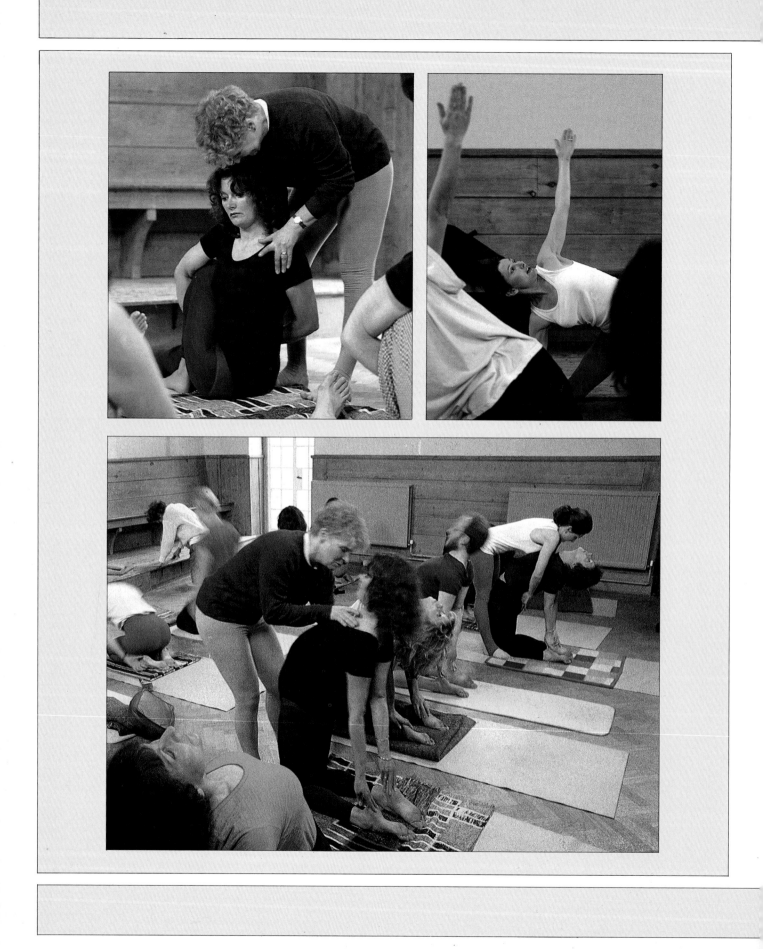

Although the stretches are graded, this does not turn the book into a ladder of excellence that you must climb. *Stretch and Relax* should be a pleasure to do, bringing a feeling of revitalized energy each time you practice. If you're elderly or stiff, you will benefit as much from the "less-stretch" movements as younger, more supple exercisers will from extending a bit farther. Anyone, from grandparent to grandchild, can practice stretching and relaxing and enjoy it.

·STRETCH·IS·NATURAL·

As you adapt to the demands of your life, you acquire tensions and stiffnesses. Even sportsmen and fitness enthusiasts seldom use the full range of their bodies' possible movements. Over the years, natural posture is pulled out of alignment by habitual muscular tensions, and your capacity for standing upright and balanced to allow free movement with minimum effort is lost. *Stretch and Relax* will help you re-align your posture and aid your natural ability to adapt to your surroundings. And it will help keep fatigue at bay. It works in harmony with your natural gifts of readjustment and recuperation, rather than imposing something alien or difficult on your body.

·RELAX·AFTER·STRETCHING·

Stretching and relaxation go together. When you stretch your body, you feel ready to relax afterward. As you concentrate on the movements and understand what you're doing, you also calm down. Relaxation is an essential part of daily life. When you practice the stretches, you begin to understand the meaning of relaxation as muscular tension releases. When you finish stretching, the natural conclusion is to lie down and give yourself a few minutes of quiet.

·BE·AWARE·OF·YOUR·BODY·

This system will help you improve your health sensibly by becoming aware of your own body and how it is constructed. It shows you how to improve your body's performance and encourages you to help yourself with minor physical and emotional problems. It is not about getting thin through exercise, and we do not include diets or arduous regimes. However, we do want you to think about your body constructively, so you feel good and look good.

We all need high levels of energy to cope with the pressures of our lives. We can all benefit from learning how to use our bodies with the maximum efficiency for the least expenditure of energy. This system will help you achieve this.

·HOW·TO·USE·THIS·BOOK·

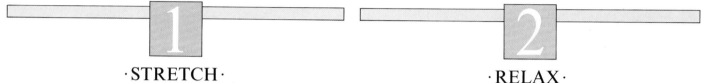

This book tells you how to stretch and relax. It will serve you
for many years if you use it properly. It is a book to work
and live with, not just to read from beginning to end.
The first three chapters are the key to the system.
The rest of the book uses the basic stretch system
for several different purposes.

1

·STRETCH·
(pages 14 to 47)

In this chapter, stretches are explained in detail.
Each basic stretch has alternatives – "less-stretch"
movements for those who are stiff or who are
beginners, "more-stretch" positions for those who
have practiced for a while and who are flexible.
Make sure you follow the precise instructions
for each stretch, especially when you first start
to practice.

2

·RELAX·
(pages 48 to 57)

Relaxation is discussed here. If you find the classic
position for relaxation described on pages 50 and
51 uncomfortable or unsuitable, there are
alternative positions on pages 52 and 53. When
you are used to relaxing, you may like to do some
deep breathing, as described on pages 54 and 55.

3

·STRETCH·PROGRAMS·
(pages 58 to 73)

This chapter combines Chapter One with Chapter
Two to give *Stretch and Relax* programs for daily
practice. Once you are completely familiar with
the stretches, use this chapter as a quick guide.
There are five different 20-minute programs, for
daily use according to your age and physical
ability. There are two longer programs for
occasional use.

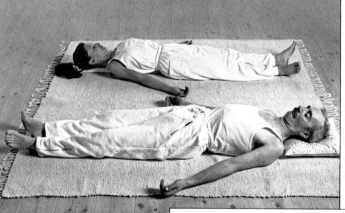

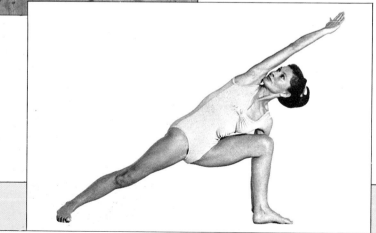

·STRETCH·TOGETHER·
(pages 74 to 89)

This is a lighthearted look at how to enjoy stretch with your family or friends. You may take turns stretching, or you can stretch together.

·RELIEVING·STIFFNESS·
(pages 90 to 113)

You may find certain stretches difficult because some part of your body is particularly stiff. Special stretches to loosen stiffness are given in this chapter. Do them daily for as long as your problem persists; practice them immediately before your regular program.

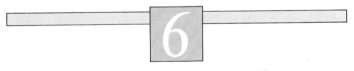

·RELIEVING·STRESS·
(pages 114 to 127)

This chapter is a little different, because it is not about regular routine. As you practice *Stretch and Relax,* you will discover extending your body can have an effect on the way you feel mentally. This chapter suggests ways to apply the technique to help you surmount crises in your life brought on by stress.

·HAVING·A·BABY·
(pages 128 to 143)

Chapter Seven can help you before, during and after birth. Stretches develop naturally from the routines covered earlier in the book.

·STRETCH·MORE·
(pages 144 to 155)

This chapter gives you a taste of what you can do after you have mastered all the stretches and programs in the book. Practice should develop over the years so it never becomes stale. Here you have a chance to see what can be achieved, preferably with the help of a teacher, by those who have practiced *Stretch and Relax* for many years and who fully understand the movements in the simpler stretches.

It is more important to develop a regular pattern of practice and to understand its effects than it is to attempt more-difficult stretches, so there is no hurry – or even need – to reach the end of the book.

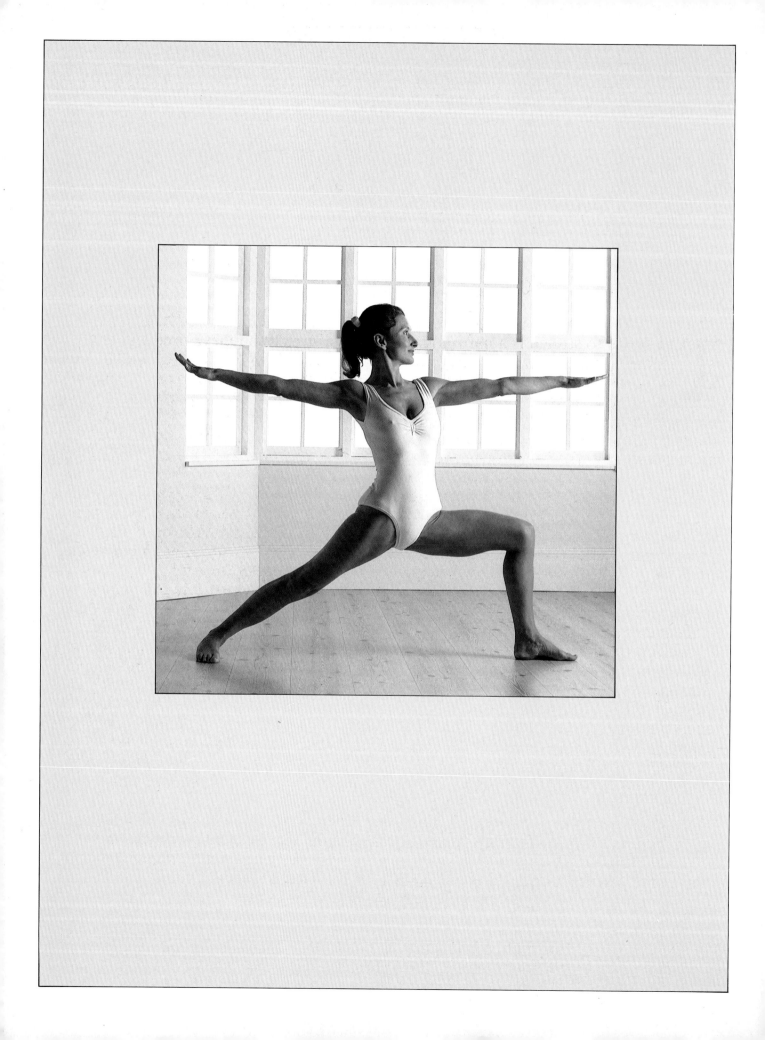

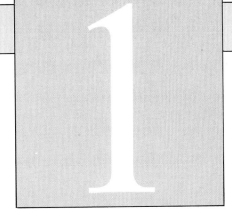

· STRETCH ·

The desire to stretch is a natural impulse – you stretch to relieve tiredness or stiffness after being in one position too long. As a form of exercise, stretching is easy, enjoyable and safe. It's the perfect antidote to physical and mental tension. Stretch is good for your entire body, especially the spine. It releases tightness in your muscles and improves circulation and relieves stress, leaving you fresh and relaxed.

By practicing regularly, you can help undo recent muscle tensions and gradually relax ones you've had for a long time, so slowly your posture and range of movement will improve.

But stretch is far more than just undoing of tension. It's the dynamic extension of the muscles. You focus your attention on the movement of your entire body; you don't just work on a particular group of muscles or a particular joint. This concentration brings insight and awareness of the way your body moves, and you'll find your physical, mental and emotional energy revived.

Breathing deeply is part of stretching. When you stretch to relieve fatigue, you may yawn at the same time, taking in a deep breath, followed by an out-breath at the end of the stretch. This link between the movement of your body and your breath is more fully developed when you stretch regularly. Don't hold your breath and breathe slowly and evenly. After awhile, correct breathing as you stretch will be automatic. Each of the seven stretches in this chapter is designed to stretch and strengthen your spine. This will energize your entire body. The order in which you practice the stretches is important. The opposing movements must counter each other, and the strong outward stretches must be balanced by more centered positions. Learn the stretches in the order they appear in this chapter, and practice each stretch *every* day. When you're familiar with them, you can put them into programs. See Chapter Three, pages 58 to 73.

The intensity of the stretch varies from one individual to the next, and it's important to understand that keeping your body supple and relaxed is not a competition.

In fact, however fit and flexible you are, start with the "less-stretch" movements to make sure you feel and understand the stretches correctly. Regularity of practice, not intensity of practice, is the key to success.

·GENERAL·POINTS·

Read the following points before you start to stretch.
They are important if you want to stretch in complete safety
and get the most out of your practice.

1 If you are healthy, you can stretch. The simple "less-stretch" variations of the basic positions should be possible for anyone to do. If you have any doubts at all, take medical advice before you start to practice.

2 Go slowly. If you decide to follow the basic program, learn the "less-stretch" positions for each stretch first, so your body gets used to the correct movements. The "more-stretch" positions demand strength and flexibility. Even if you do other forms of physical exercise and your body is already very flexible when you start stretching, practice the basic stretches daily for some months before you try anything more advanced.

3 Practice the stretches in the order they are presented. Learn them in sequence; do not pick out one or two in isolation.

4 In many of these positions you keep your legs straight. To prevent yourself from pushing into the backs of your knees and injuring your ligaments, pull up your kneecaps by tightening your front thigh muscles. Extend the lower back and keep the abdominal muscles firm.

5 Wear loose clothing, whatever feels comfortable. Leotards and tights are not essential.

6 Work on a non-slip surface with bare feet so you can stretch your toes for maximum contact with the floor.

7 Do not practice immediately after eating.

8 Rest when your body is tired. Your stamina will increase as you practice regularly.

9 Relax your muscles and never force your body into a stretch. As you extend your limbs, your muscles elongate away from your spine, enabling your joints to move freely.

10 Go into each movement on an out-breath and then breathe normally. Do not hold your breath, as this causes tension and strain. Breathe out on exertion. As you come up out of the stretch, breathe in.

11 Jump your feet into position, when you need to take them wide apart. If you are pregnant or elderly, it's probably more sensible to step into position. The instructions suggest how far apart you should take your feet. These distances are only approximate and may be varied according to your height.

12 Hold each stretch as long as you can comfortably continue releasing your muscles. At first this will be only a few seconds, but as you begin to practice regularly the time you hold a stretch will gradually increase.

13 Be aware of the way your spine moves as you stretch. Feel the movement along the back of your body as well as the front. If this is difficult, ask someone to help you with a pole. See Chapter Four, pages 74 to 89.

14 Do each side stretch on both sides, holding the position on the second side the same length of time as on the first. You may find you stretch more on your stronger side; make sure you work on both sides evenly. Stretch on your non-preferred side first.

15 Come up out of the positions with as much care as you go into them. To come out of a stretch, repeat the movements you used to go into it, in reverse order. Take especial care with the upside-down positions (see pages 42 to 47), because coming out of them too fast could put excessive strain on the vertebrae of the neck.

·STRAIGHT·

Stretching your spine up, against the pull of gravity, allows your entire body to move freely and easily. Follow the instructions below, and you'll feel the benefits as you do the outward stretches.

Start from your feet
Stand with the outer edges of your bare feet parallel to each other and your big toes touching. You may have to keep heels slightly apart. Stretch your toes fully to help balance you and support your trunk. (If you have bunions or deformed toes, you may find this difficult – see pages 112 and 113.) From the balls of your feet, extend back into your heels. Your weight should be distributed evenly on the arches of both feet, and you should feel firm and stable on the floor.

Lift from your arches, and stretch up through your legs. Pull up your kneecaps by tightening your front thigh muscles. The backs of your knees should also extend, but don't push back into them; this could strain your calf muscles. Tighten the muscles underneath your buttocks so your tailbone feels "tucked in." When held correctly, the pelvis is horizontal, not tilted backward or forward (see page 93). In this position, it gives the spine maximum support.

Stretch up through your spine
As you stretch up from your pelvis, the muscles of your abdomen help your lumbar spine extend and keep it from sagging in. This relieves pressure on your lower back. Lift your ribcage at the back and front, and feel muscles of the back of the chest stretch away from your spine. This is called *opening the chest*. Make space between your hips and your ribs.

Stretch your arms above your head, feeling the lift in your spine. Then drop them by your side, without losing the spinal stretch. Drop your shoulders. Relax them while maintaining the lift in your spine. Hold your arms loosely, and use their weight to help your shoulders drop.

Extend your neck up into the base of your skull without lifting your chin or pulling it in too far. You want to feel as if you are being pulled up by the crown of your head. Your entire body should feel firm, but light, while you breathe smoothly and easily.

From this basic standing stretch, your body is free to move in all directions.

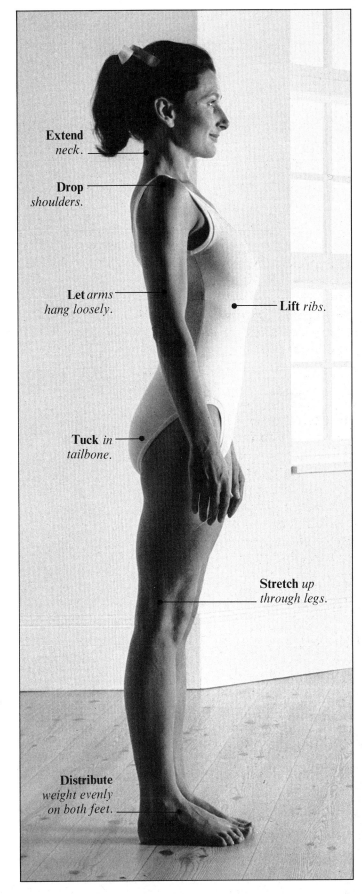

Extend *neck.*

Drop *shoulders.*

Let *arms hang loosely.*

Lift *ribs.*

Tuck *in tailbone.*

Stretch *up through legs.*

Distribute *weight evenly on both feet.*

·SIDEWAYS·

In these stretches you extend the entire spine to the side, keeping your hips and spine flexible. It is a movement you should practice regularly because as you get older you are unlikely to move like this very often in your daily activities.

The firm stretch of the legs allows the lower spine to release, which relieves lower backache. The outstretched arms and the extension of the back of the neck keep the upper spine mobile.

If your hips are stiff when you start to practice, you may try to go down too far, and bend from the waist instead of the hips. Your trunk will drop forward, and you will lose the sideways stretch in the lower back. In order to get used to the correct stretch in the hips and lower back, first practice the "less stretch" positions on page 20. Exercises on page 78 also help you with the correct alignment of this position.

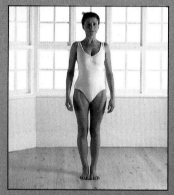

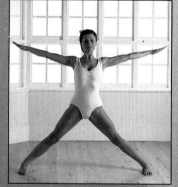

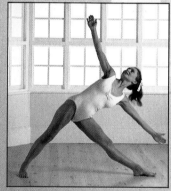

1 Stand tall, and stretch up through your spine. With feet together, spread out your toes and pull up from your arches. Pull up your kneecaps, and stretch your entire spine. Extend your neck, and relax your face.

2 Spread your feet 36 inches apart, keeping them parallel. Maintain the lift of your spine so your chest is open, and your shoulders are relaxed. Stretch out your arms, with the palms of your hands facing the floor.

3 Turn your right foot slightly in and your left leg out to the side. Line up your left heel with the arch of your right foot. Pull up your kneecaps. Breathing out, move your hips to the right, and extend your spine sideways to the left.

Pull *up kneecaps, and keep back-leg strong.*

Stretch *into fingertips, and make sure palms of hands are facing forward.*

Keep *upper arm in line with lower arm.*

Extend *lower back.*

Make sure *chest is open, and keep it facing forward.*

4 Keep your tailbone well tucked under. Tighten the muscles underneath your buttocks, and stretch sideways until your left hand rests behind your left leg. Turn your head, and look up at your outstretched fingers. Breathe normally. Hold the position for up to 30 seconds. Breathe in as you come up, then repeat on the other side.

Be sure *heel is in line with arch of right foot.*

·SIDEWAYS·
LESS STRETCH

The stiffer you are, the more important it is to get a good stretch *before* you go sideways. Stretches on this page help release stiffness, especially in the hips. If you have the sensation of dropping forward, practice with your back against a wall.

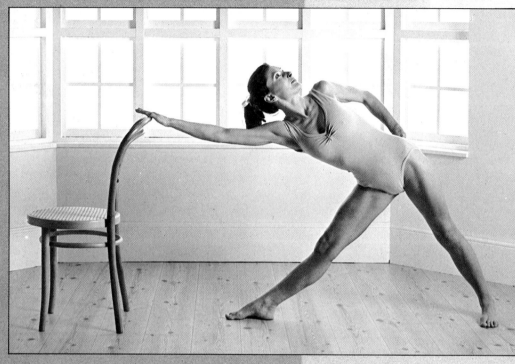

First stretch
Place a chair to your right. Spread your feet about 36 inches apart, and stretch your arms out. Turn your left foot slightly in and your right leg out, as shown on pages 18 and 19. Put your left hand on your hip, and stretch to the right. Stretch your lower spine. Hold for a few seconds. Breathe in as you come up, and repeat on the other side.

Second stretch
Stand tall, and stretch up through your spine. Spread your feet 36 inches apart, and stretch out your arms. Turn your left foot slightly in and your right leg out. Breathe out. Put your right hand on your leg, and stretch to the right without bending forward. Hold for a few seconds. Breathe in as you come up, and repeat on the other side.

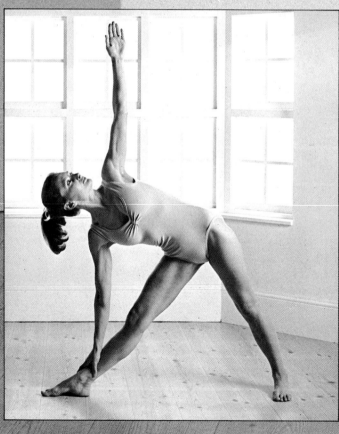

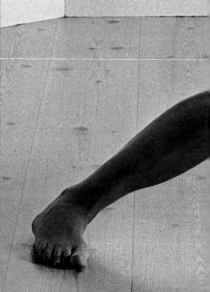

·SIDEWAYS·
MORE STRETCH

This exhilarating stretch increases flexibility in the hips and spine, and tones the muscles in the abdomen and legs. The intense stretch along the upper side of the body loosens the shoulders while the expansion in the chest is good for breathing.

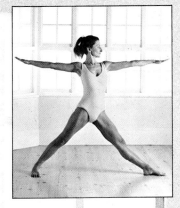

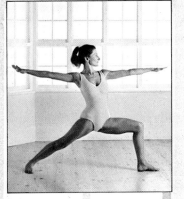

1 Spread your feet as far apart as is comfortable for you (about 54 inches). Turn your right foot in and your left leg out to the side. Turn your left thigh out at the hip, and pull up your kneecaps.

2 Keep your right leg firm while you bend your left knee to a right angle. Do this by lowering your hips so your left thigh is parallel to the floor.

3 Breathe out, and extend your trunk along your left thigh. Take your left hand down behind your foot, and press your left knee back against your armpit. Stretch your right arm over your right ear. Extend your spine to the left. Keep your right shoulder back, and look up. Breathe normally as you hold for 20 seconds. Breathe in as you come up, and repeat on the other side.

·WIDE & STRONG·

These strong, dynamic stretches extend the limbs away from the center of the body and stretch the spine. They loosen the hip joints and tone leg muscles. They are very good for athletic people, especially runners. Invigorating stretches such as these need stability, so feet should be firm and strong on the floor. Your spine lifts as your arms stretch powerfully, and your breath deepens as your chest expands. At first you may be able to hold the stretch comfortably for only a short time, but with continued practice your stamina will increase.

If your hips and shoulders are stiff, practice the "less-stretch" positions on page 24 until you feel able to do the fuller stretches.

Extend *back arm strongly.*

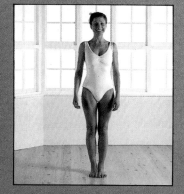

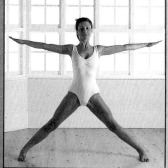

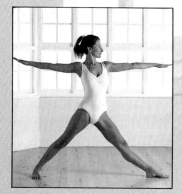

1 Stand tall and straight with feet together. Press your feet firmly into the floor. Pull up from your arches. Stretch up through your legs and along the curves of your spine. Keep shoulders down and facial muscles completely relaxed.

2 Spread your feet as far apart as is comfortable for you (about 54 inches). Keep the upward stretch in your spine, and extend your arms at shoulder level. Stretch away from your trunk into your fingertips. The palms of your hands face the floor.

3 Turn your right foot slightly in and your left leg out. Align your left heel with the arch of your right foot. Turn your head to the left, and keep the stretch wide and strong. Focus your eyes beyond your fingertips, and try to keep your shoulders relaxed.

4 Breathing out, bend your left knee and take your hips down. Your left thigh is parallel to the floor, with a right angle at the knee. Keep your right leg straight, and stretch out strongly from the center. Hold for up to 30 seconds. Breathe in as you come up, and repeat on the other side.

Keep *outside of back foot on floor.*

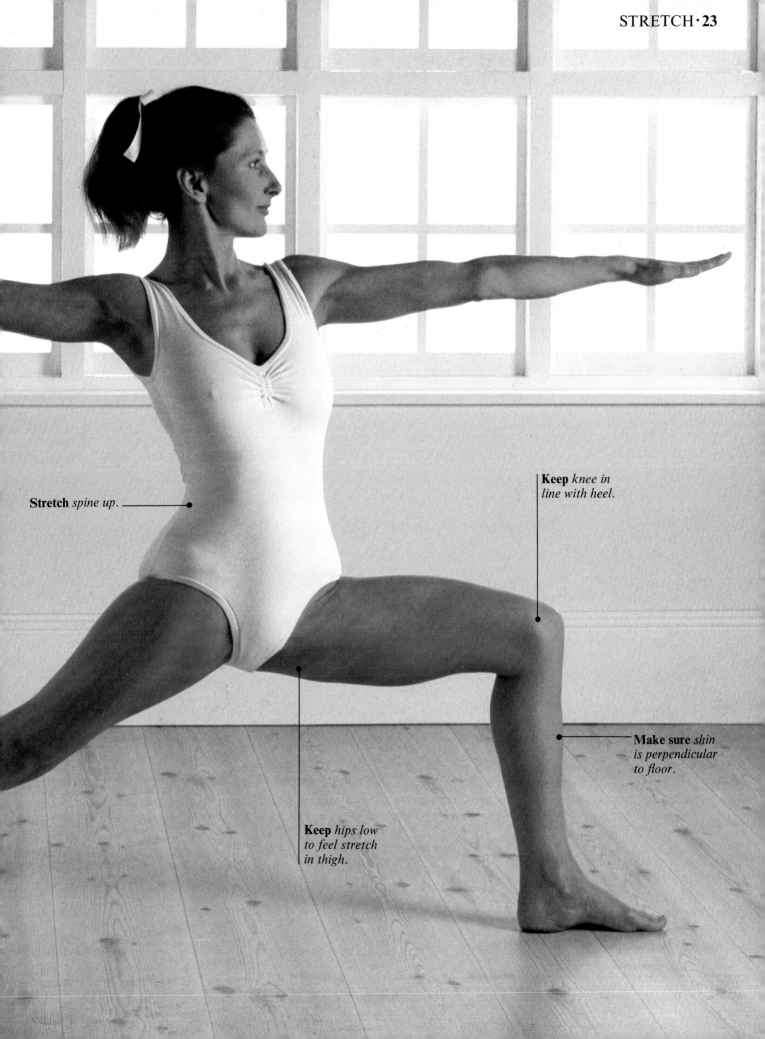

Keep *knee in line with heel.*

Stretch *spine up.*

Make sure *shin is perpendicular to floor.*

Keep *hips low to feel stretch in thigh.*

·WIDE & STRONG·
LESS STRETCH

With age your shoulder joints stiffen, making it hard to extend the body as a whole. The stretches on this page help keep shoulder joints flexible, while the upward stretch of the arms lifts the spine.

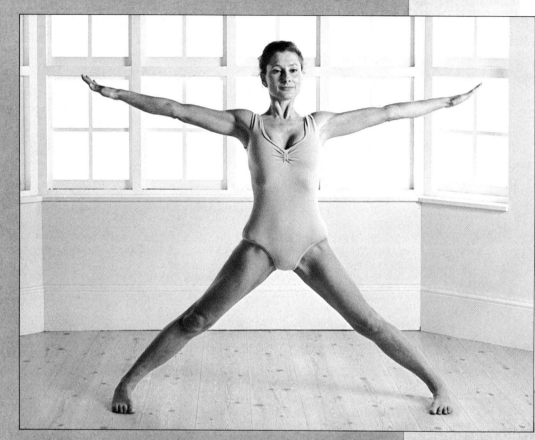

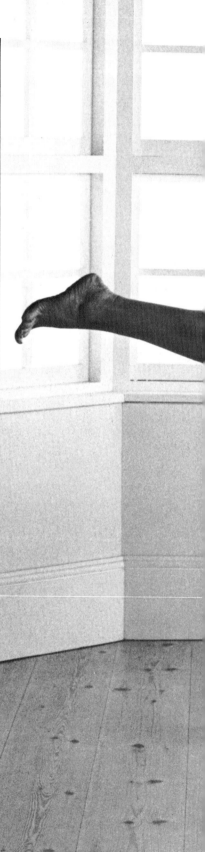

First stretch
Spread your feet wide apart, with your toes pointing forward and arches of your feet lifted up. Turn your thighs outward, and keep knees straight. Stretch your arms from your spine into your fingertips. Your breathing will deepen as your chest expands. Hold for a few seconds.

Second stretch
Stretch your arms out as described above. Breathing out, stretch your arms above your head. Your palms face each other. Keep the outsides of your feet firmly on the floor. Take a few deep breaths, and stretch up each time you breathe out, then lower arms.

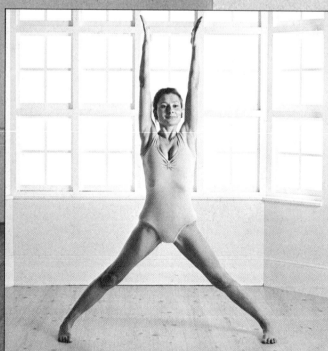

·WIDE & STRONG·
MORE STRETCH

These advanced stretches require strong back muscles and flexible hips and shoulders. You may find it difficult to balance in the second stretch; if so practice only the first position until you gain confidence. Then you will feel able to balance securely on one leg.

First stretch

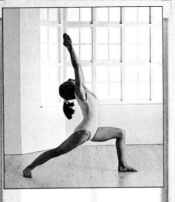

Stand with your feet wide apart. Point your right foot in and your left leg out. Turn completely to the left, and stretch your arms up over your head, with palms facing each other. Lift your back ribs as you stretch into your fingertips. Breathing out, bend your left knee, and lower your hips until your left leg is at a right angle to your knee. Breathe normally for up to 20 seconds. Breathe in as you come up, and repeat on the other side.

Second stretch

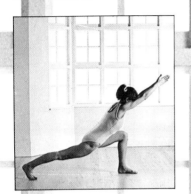

1 Proceed from the last stretch by lifting your back heel, tucking in your tailbone and stretching forward along your front thigh. Keep hips down so your lower back is extended.

2 Breathe in, and reach forward. As you lift your back foot, breathe out and straighten your left leg. Keep arms and wrists firmly stretched as you extend your body. There should be a straight line from the fingertips to the heel. Hold for a few seconds. Come down, and repeat on the other side.

·BACK·TO·THE·CENTER·

As you do these stretches, your limbs are brought back to the center of your body after the strong outward movements. This helps you concentrate and gives a feeling of calmness.

Be careful to maintain the upward lift of the spine, or you will lose the energizing effect of the outward stretches. Keep your eyes open, and look forward without straining.

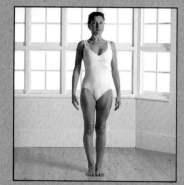

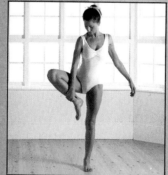

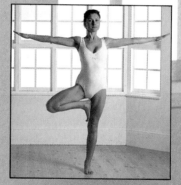

1 Stand up tall and straight, with feet together. Pull up through your legs, and stretch along the curves of your spine. Keep your tailbone tucked in and shoulders relaxed.

2 Bend your right knee, and use one or both hands to raise your right leg. Place your right foot as high as possible on the inside of your left thigh, so toes are pointing down.

3 Extend your arms at shoulder level, and stretch into your fingertips. To help you balance, keep your left leg straight and strong, and spread the toes of your left foot. Extend your lower back and keep the abdominal muscles firm. You should feel firm as you balance on one leg.

4 Keep your spine straight and your shoulders relaxed. Open your chest, and bring your palms together. Your right foot should press on your inside left thigh, while your left leg stays straight and stable. Take a few deep breaths, repeat on the other side.

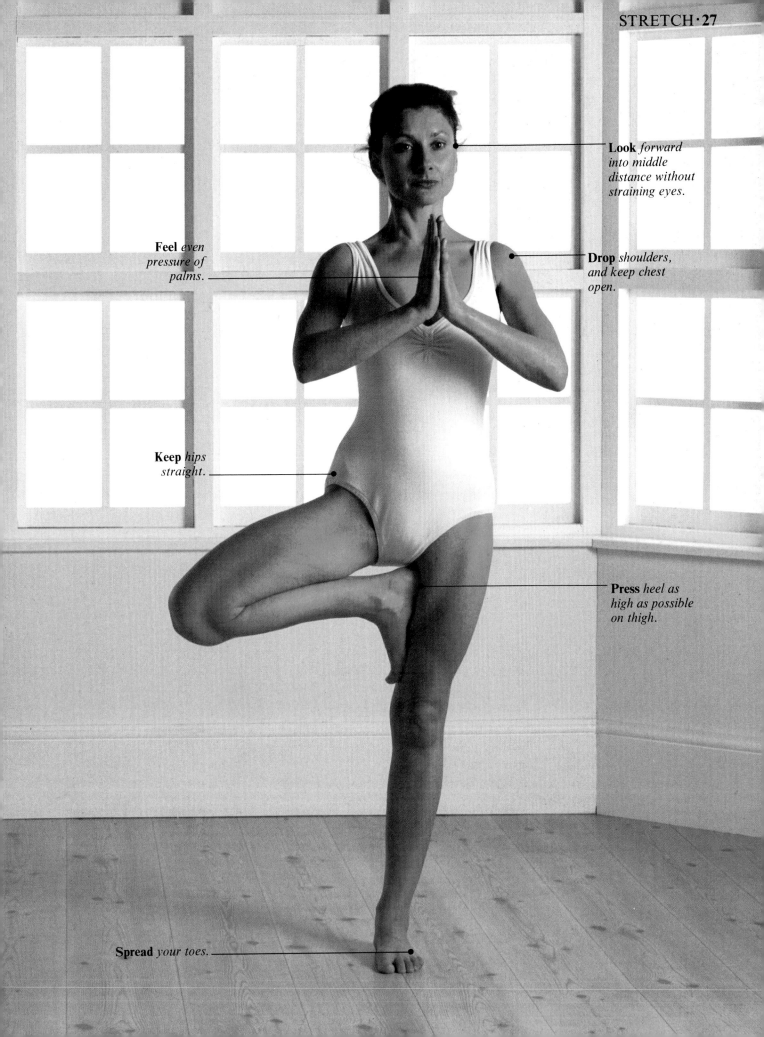

Look *forward into middle distance without straining eyes.*

Feel *even pressure of palms.*

Drop *shoulders, and keep chest open.*

Keep *hips straight.*

Press *heel as high as possible on thigh.*

Spread *your toes.*

·BACK·TO·THE·CENTER·
LESS STRETCH

You may find it difficult to balance steadily on one leg in the basic stretch position when you begin. If so, practice the positions on this page for a few months. They improve flexibility in the hips, and they have a calming effect.

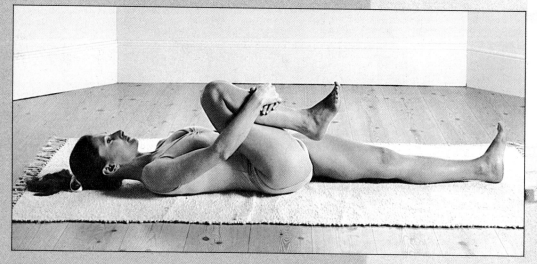

First stretch

Lie down on your back on a rug. Breathing out, bend your right leg, and bring it close to your trunk. Keep your left leg straight, and gently pull your right leg toward you until you can grasp the shin. Your hips should stay flat on the floor. Hold for 30 seconds, and repeat on the other side.

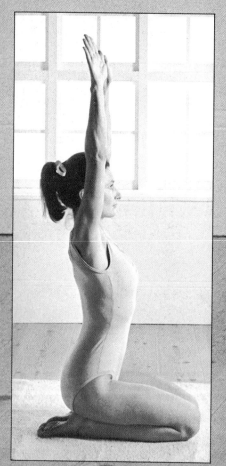

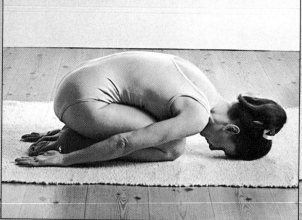

Second stretch

1 Kneel on a thick soft rug or blanket on the floor, sitting on your heels. Link your fingers together, turn your palms outward and stretch your arms up over your head. Release fingers. Keep your bottom down on your heels.

2 Bring your arms down close to your thighs, and fold your body forward. Lower your head until it touches the ground. Breathe out as you bend forward and breathe naturally for about 1 minute. Breathe in, as you uncurl slowly and come up. Repeat the stretch starting with your fingers linked and the opposite thumb on top.

·BACK·TO·THE·CENTER·
MORE STRETCH

This position is difficult because you need to turn the thighs out at the hips and stretch up at the same time. Most people will have to practice this for many months before they feel comfortable.

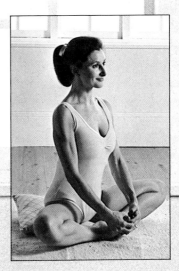

Stretch
Sit on the floor with your legs straight out in front of you. Stretch up with arms behind you and fingers touching the floor. Spread your legs wide, then bend your knees. Bring your feet close to your body, with soles together. Your thighs should turn out and your knees go down. (See photo at left.) If it is hard to keep your lower back stretching up, raise your hips by sitting on a cushion. (See photo above.) Hold your feet with your hands, and stretch along your spine. Relax your hips more so your knees go down more. Hold for up to 60 seconds.

·FORWARD·

These stretches are very good for the lower back when done correctly. The problem is the pelvis needs to rotate forward around the top of the thigh bones if the trunk is to move forward freely. Many people find the correct rotation hard and compensate by putting extra strain on the spine. If tight back-thigh muscles (hamstrings) make correct rotation difficult, practice for several months the positions shown on page 32.

Stand or sit with weight evenly distributed, and make sure you are straight. Always remember the movement is *up* and forward. Stretch away from your hips, and keep your chest open so you can breathe naturally through the stretch. If you have a slipped disk or lumbago (see pages 96 to 99), do not practice the bending part of these stretches. Practice the upward-forward movements only.

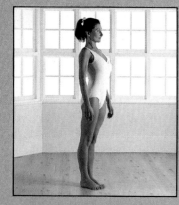

1 Stand tall and straight, with feet together. Pull up through your legs, and stretch along the length of your spine. Make your neck long, and keep your shoulders and arms relaxed.

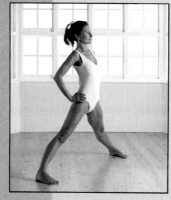

2 Spread your feet very wide apart. Keep toes pointing forward and your arches lifted up. Bend your elbows, and put your hands on your hips. Lifting from the hips, stretch up through your spine.

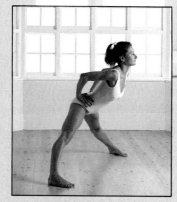

3 Keeping your legs straight, breathe out, and stretch forward from the hips. Do not push into the back of your knees. Keep your back extended and your body weight evenly supported by your feet.

4 Continue to stretch forward until you can place your hands on the floor in front of you. Pull up the back of your thighs, and extend the front of your trunk forward and upward.

Keep *weight on feet, and press them firmly into the ground.*

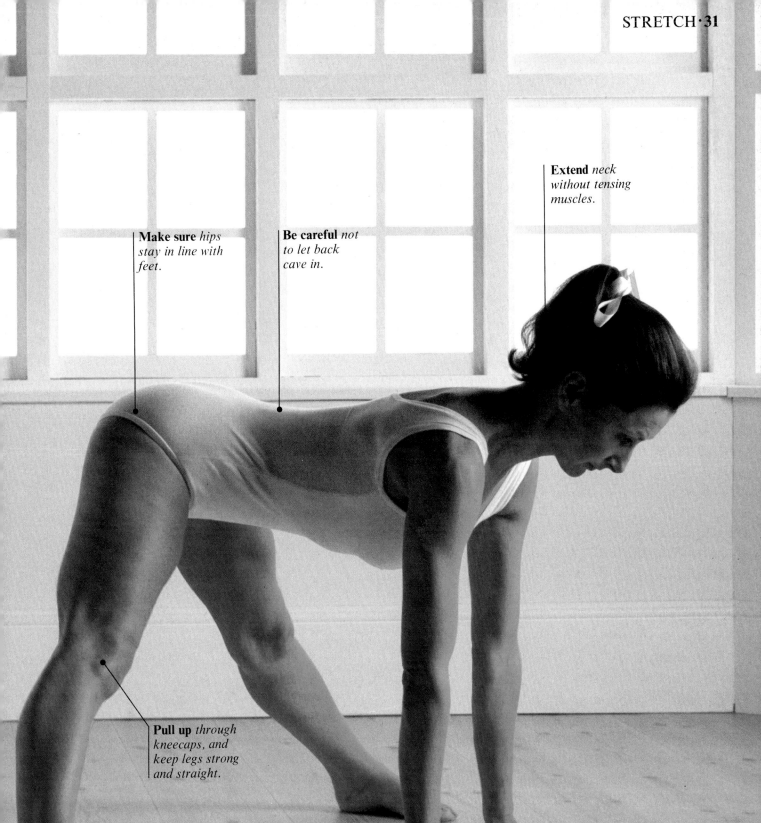

Extend *neck without tensing muscles.*

Make sure *hips stay in line with feet.*

Be careful *not to let back cave in.*

Pull up *through kneecaps, and keep legs strong and straight.*

Keep *hands shoulder-width apart.*

·FORWARD·
LESS STRETCH

When you bend forward, you have to bend from the hips and your spine. These "less-stretch" positions are for people who have tight hamstrings that keep the pelvis from rotating forward over the tops of the thigh bones.

First stretch
Put a chair against the wall so it cannot slip. Stand facing it, so when you go forward you will touch the chair back. Your feet should be about 12 inches apart and parallel. Keeping your legs straight, stretch up and forward from your hips. Put your hands on the back of the chair. Breathing out, extend the stretch as far as you can. Lengthen the front of your body, and keep your back straight. Your hips should stay in line with your feet. You will feel the stretch in the back of your thighs. Hold the position for up to 30 seconds. Breathe in as you come up.

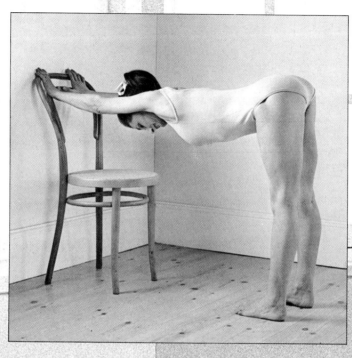

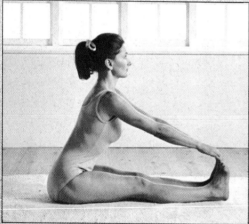

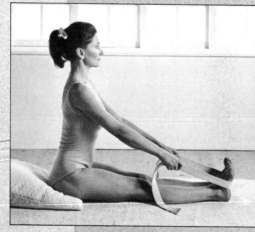

Second stretch
Sit on the floor with your legs straight out in front of you. Your weight should be a little to the front of your buttock bones so you can lift from your lower back. If this is difficult, sit on a cushion or folded blanket. Stretch up and forward so you can catch your feet. (See photo above left.) If you collapse at your waist when you do this, loop a belt or necktie around your feet and hold that. (See photo above right.) Your legs should stay straight. If they bend, use the belt. Move from the base of your spine, and do not pull hard with your hands. Elongate the back of your neck, and keep shoulders relaxed. Hold for as long as you can without strain or tightness (up to 30 seconds). Breathe normally. Do not practice the basic stretch until you can do this without the belt.

·FORWARD·
MORE STRETCH

When the pelvis rotates forward correctly, you can bend without putting undue strain on your lumbar spine. In these positions you should be able to stretch forward without straining or pulling with your hands.

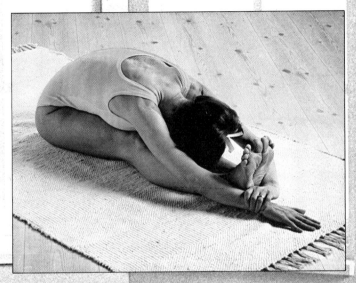

First stretch
Sit on the floor, and catch your feet as in the "less-stretch" position opposite. Breathing out, stretch the front of your trunk forward along your thighs. Do not pull with your hands but extend gently from the base of your spine. Lower your head. Eventually you will be able to hold your hands beyond the soles of your feet and let your shoulders relax. Stay in this position for up to 30 seconds while breathing normally. Then sit up as you breathe in. This is a good alternative to the standing stretch. (See photo at left.)

Second stretch
Try this stretch only if the back of your thighs extend without strain and you can put your hands on the floor keeping your knees straight. Do not hyperextend your legs. Stand with your feet together and your legs straight. Raise your arms above your head, and stretch up tall. Bring your arms down, and bend forward while breathing out. Extending your spine and keeping your lower back concave for as long as possible, relax your neck. Continue to bend forward from your hips. The top of your head should move toward your feet. If you are supple, you will be able to hold your hands behind your ankles. Stay in the position, and breathe normally. Then come up. Breathing in, extend forward. Breathe out, and stand straight.

·TWIST·

Twisting positions keep the spine flexible and help release tension in the hips and shoulders. When the movements are done correctly, shoulders move back and down, and the top of the spine moves in. This is an excellent stretch for correcting a rounded back. See page 99.

The thoracic vertebrae of the upper back rotate more freely than the large lumbar vertebrae of the waist. So it is important to stretch properly from the lower back. Turn the spine completely as you twist; do not just push the chest out and turn the ribcage. Because of the upward-inward movement of the lower back, twisting positions are good for lower back pain.

The correct movements can be hard to understand, so start with the "less-stretch" positions, however supple you are. Your aim is to rotate your body around your straight spine as you stretch up.

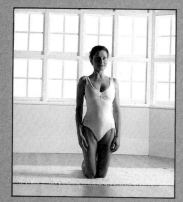 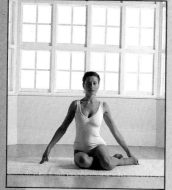 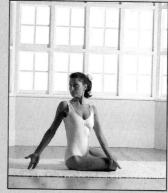

1 Kneel with your knees and feet together. Stretch up along the curves of your spine, keeping your shoulders down. Extend your neck, and let your arms relax.

2 Slide your hips to the right, and sit on the floor with your legs folded behind you to the left. Keep your left buttock on the ground. If this is difficult, sit on a small cushion. Lift from your lower back and stretch upward through the crown of your head.

3 Place your left hand on the outside of your right knee. Place your right arm behind you. Breathing out, twist around as far as you can to the right, without raising your left hip. Keep your right knee in line with your hip. Keep fingertips of your right hand on the floor.

4 When you can get a good twist, hold the back of your left arm with your right hand. Breathing normally, hold the position for 30 seconds. Relax, then repeat on the other side.

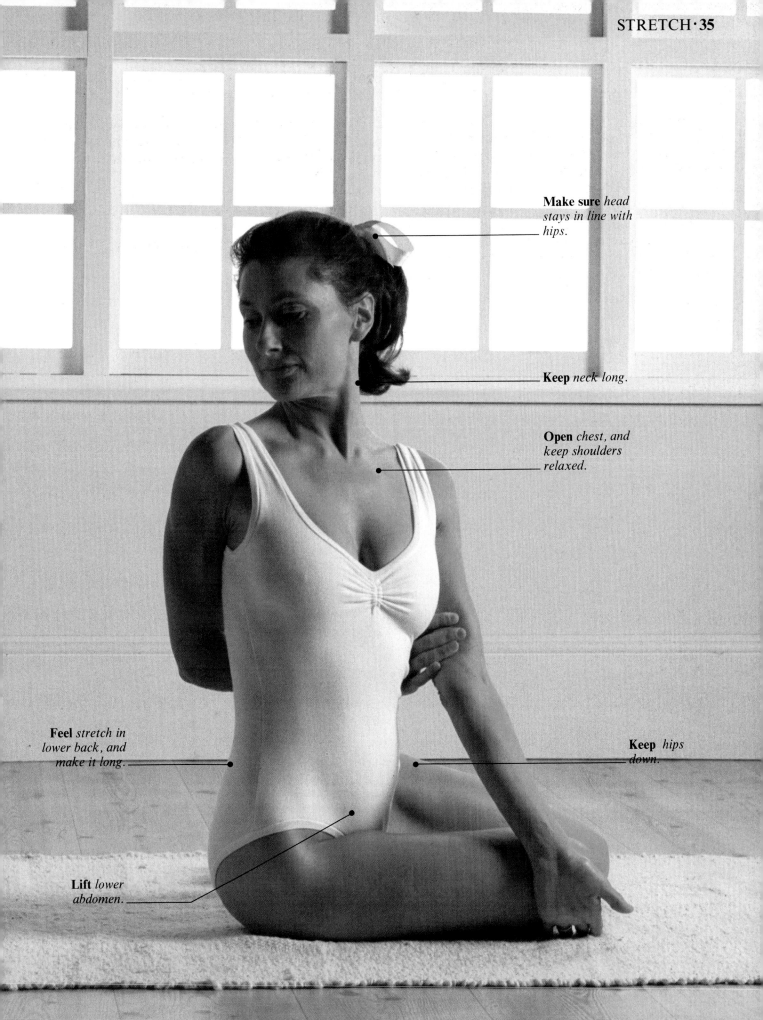

Make sure *head stays in line with hips.*

Keep *neck long.*

Open *chest, and keep shoulders relaxed.*

Feel *stretch in lower back, and make it long.*

Keep *hips down.*

Lift *lower abdomen.*

·TWIST·
LESS STRETCH

The stretches on this page are beneficial if you have stiff joints or if you stoop. They are particularly useful if you cannot sit in the basic position on pages 34 and 35, or if you find it difficult to lift your lower back.

First stretch
Sit on a chair with weight slightly forward. Do not collapse the back of your waist, but sit up tall, so the front of your body is stretched and your chest is open. Without moving your hips, twist to the right, and hold the back of the chair seat with your right hand. Put the back of your left hand against your right thigh. Keep your knees in line with your hips. As you turn, drop your shoulders, and let your spine stretch up from the hips. Hold for 30 seconds. Relax and repeat on the other side.

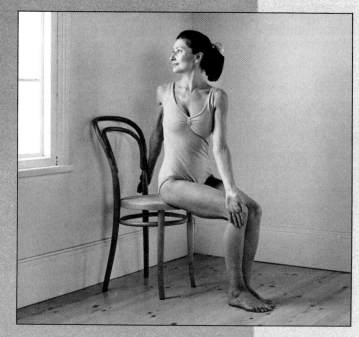

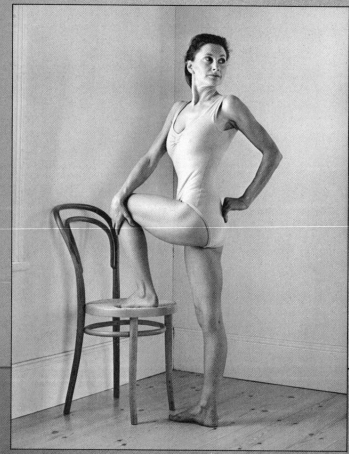

Second stretch
Stand facing a chair, with your feet pointing straight ahead. Put your left foot on the seat. Keep your left hip down. If you are very tall, you may have to put a book on the seat of the chair. Stand up tall, and extend the front of your body, keeping your shoulders down and your chest open. Put your left hand on the base of your spine. Put your right hand against your left thigh. Without moving your hips, twist as far around to the left as you can. Look back over your left shoulder. Hold for 30 seconds. Relax and repeat on the other side.

·TWIST·
MORE STRETCH

In these twists you must feel the movement in your lower back. You must stretch the spine as you start to turn, while keeping it elongated. Because this is difficult when you are sitting with legs straight out in front of you, do not attempt the second stretch on this page unless you can easily do the "more stretch forward" positions on page 33.

First stretch

Stand with your feet 36 inches apart and your arms extended. Turn both feet to the left as for the "basic stretch sideways" position. See pages 18 and 19. Breathe out, and turn from your hips, extending your right arm over your left foot. Keep knees straight, and do not hyperextend your legs. Open your chest as you stretch your left arm up and out from your trunk. Turn your head to look up at your left hand. Breathing normally, hold the position for as long as you comfortably can. Then come up, and repeat on the other side.

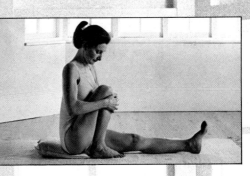

Second stretch

1 Sit with legs straight. Bend your right leg, so your heel is close to your buttock.

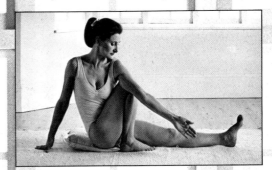

2 With your right hand on the floor behind you, lift up your ribcage so your lower back goes in. Turn as far as possible to the right. Without tensing abdominal muscles, extend the back of your left arm around the outside of your right knee.

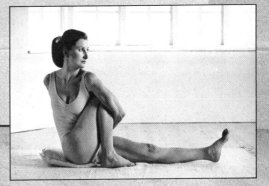

3 Clasp your hands behind your back as you turn more. Keep the outside of your right hip down. Hold for up to 20 seconds. Relax and repeat on the other side.

·BACKWARD·

The backward stretch of the spine is a powerful, invigorating movement. Because extension of the spine works directly on its natural curves, it is important not merely to exaggerate the curve at the waist and neck. Instead try to stretch the spine as a single unit, lengthening the curves and opening the chest and hips. This pose corrects rounded shoulders and prevents the convex curve of the upper spine from becoming too exaggerated. See page 99. When done properly, this stretch is the key to youthful posture and vitality.

To extend the spine evenly, strong muscles are needed as well as flexible joints. If you are very flexible, it is essential to gain strength by practicing the "less-stretch" positions described on page 40 before you attempt the more difficult backward stretches. If you are uncomfortable with your head back in the basic position, because of stiffness in the upper back and neck, practice the "less-stretch" positions first.

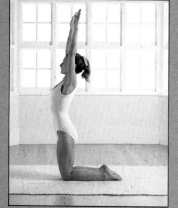

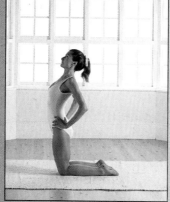

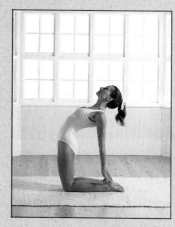

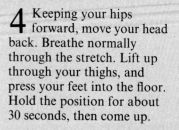

1 Kneel with your feet and knees together and weight evenly distributed. Stretch your arms above your head to lift your spine and back ribs.

2 Move your hands to your hips, and continue to stretch up. Keep the back of your waist long. As you begin to curve your spine backward, it is essential to lift and open your chest.

3 Tighten muscles underneath your buttocks, and push your hips forward so your thighs remain perpendicular. Stretch your spine in one continuous movement, and move your hands back to your heels.

4 Keeping your hips forward, move your head back. Breathe normally through the stretch. Lift up through your thighs, and press your feet into the floor. Hold the position for about 30 seconds, then come up.

Relax *and let back of neck extend.*

Keep *chest open, and breathe normally.*

Lift *upper back without tensing throat and neck.*

Push *hips forward, stretch up through thighs and tighten muscles under buttocks.*

·BACKWARD·
LESS STRETCH

Before you try the basic position, you need strong back muscles and a good extension at the hips, or you will feel constriction at the back of your waist. Do these stretches with your spine long and your chest open.

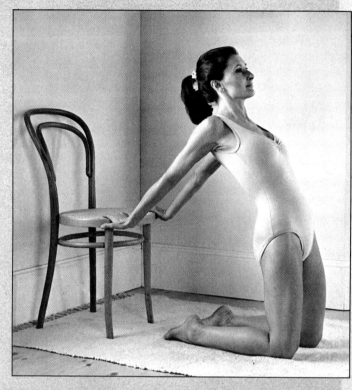

First stretch
Put a strong chair against the wall so it cannot slip. You can also use the edge of a sofa or bed. Kneel down with your back to it. Sitting on your heels, bring your hands back, and grasp the chair firmly. Push against the chair so you lift your hips away from your heels. Tighten the muscles underneath your buttocks, and bring your shoulders back. Take your thighs as far forward as possible. Lift your chest up from your hips, getting as much curve in your spine as you can. Lengthen your neck, and keep looking forward.

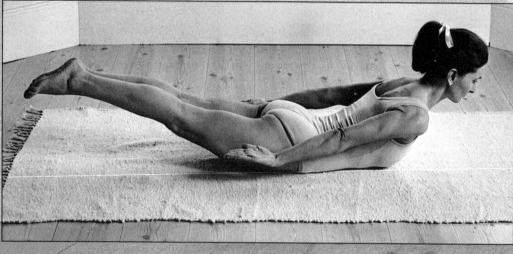

Second stretch
Lie on your front on a rug or blanket with arms down by your side and palms facing the ceiling. Stretch your legs back, and tighten the muscles underneath your buttocks. Breathe out, and lift your legs and shoulders off the floor. Keep your knees straight. The entire spine must stretch, so do not take your head higher than your feet. If your neck is stiff, extend the base of your skull away from your shoulders. Breathe normally for a few seconds, then lower your feet and head. Rest.

·BACKWARD·
MORE STRETCH

Pushing against the floor with your hands increases the intensity of this stretch, so do not try the positions on this page until you have toned your back muscles in the "less-stretch" and basic positions.

First stretch
Lie on your stomach with hands under your chest, fingers pointing forward. Tighten the muscles underneath your buttocks. Breathing out, push down with your hands and the tops of your feet, and lift your trunk and legs off the floor. Extend your spine, and straighten your arms. Keep heels together. Your weight should be taken by your hands and the tops of your feet. Breathing normally, hold for a few seconds, then come down.

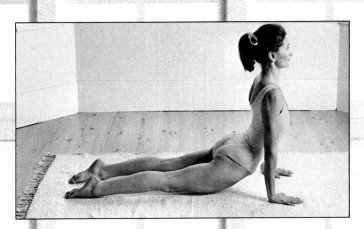

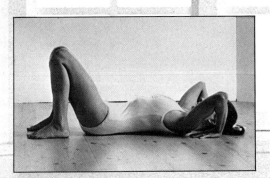

Second stretch
Don't try this stretch until you can comfortably do all the other stretches described from page 18 to 47.

1 Lie on your back, and stretch your arms over your head. Bend your knees, and bring your heels close to your buttocks, keeping your feet parallel. Put the palms of your hands under your shoulders with fingers pointing toward your feet.

2 Tuck in your tailbone, and raise your hips. As you breathe out, push your hands and feet against the floor and come up, curving your chest as you do so. Straighten your arms, and arch your back, without letting your feet and knees splay out. Come up as far as you can. Each time you breathe out, stretch farther into the back arch. Hold the position for a few breaths, then come down gently.

·UPSIDE DOWN·

Inverted positions are held for longer than the other stretches and provide a refreshing, revitalizing end to a practice session. They also promote mental relaxation. For benefits to be fully appreciated, your spine must be properly extended, so your chest is open, and breathing becomes smooth and easy.

When you start practicing, stiffness in the upper back may prevent you from placing your weight high enough on the shoulders for the full spinal stretch. Only your shoulders, upper arms and the back of your head should touch the floor.

There should be no undue pressure on your neck. Your chin should rest between your collarbones as the back of your neck stretches. If you feel your head is crooked, come down to straighten it. Practice will gradually make the positions easier, and the longer you hold them the more refreshed you will feel.

Caution: If you are menstruating or suffer from a specific medical condition, consult your doctor before doing the upside-down stretches. Instead, finish the practice session by repeating the appropriate stretches on pages 26 to 29.

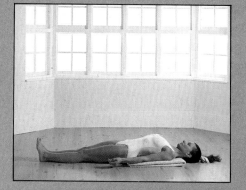

1 Lie face upward with a folded blanket under your back. If you are a beginner or have stiff shoulders, put an extra thickness of blanket under your shoulders to protect your neck.

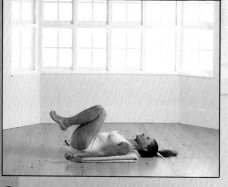

2 Press your hands against the floor. Keep your shoulders down and your chest open. Bend your knees, and raise your legs over your waist. Take two or three deep breaths.

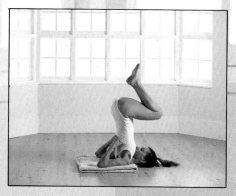

3 Pushing your palms against the floor, swing your knees up and over your head. You will feel the stretch in your upper back. Keep your arms close to your body. Bend your elbows, and support your back with your hands, with fingers spread horizontally.

Keep elbows close to each other.

Stretch *into toes.*

Make *body a straight line from ankles to shoulders.*

4 Straighten your legs, and pull them up from your hips until they are aligned with your chest. Your entire spine should stretch straight toward the ceiling. Let your throat and face relax. Hold the stretch for as long as you feel comfortable, up to 30 minutes.

To come down, bend your knees while still supporting your upper back with your hands. Uncurl your spine until you are lying flat.

Spread *fingers horizontally.*

Bring *upper back in, and stretch up.*

Let *throat and face relax, and avoid building tension in neck.*

·UPSIDE DOWN·
LESS STRETCH

If you are very stiff, you may find it difficult to swing your hips over your head in the basic position. This less-demanding variation can be done with a chair, as shown here, or with your feet pushing against a wall. Make sure you cannot slide as you push with your feet.

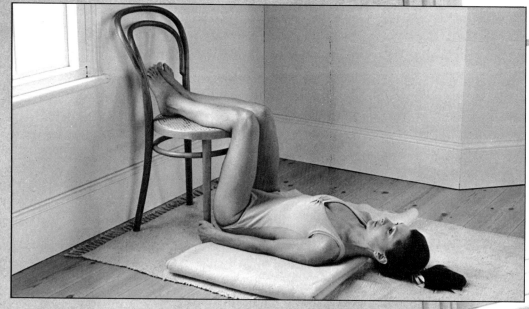

1 Place a chair against a wall. Lie on your back, a thick blanket under your shoulders, your knees bent and your legs comfortably supported on the chair. Hold the legs of the chair. Alternative position: Omit the chair, and adopt the same position with your hips lying close to the wall. Push your feet against the wall, and keep palms flat on the ground.

2 Slide feet along the seat of the chair, and push against it with your feet. Hold on to the chair legs. Tighten your buttocks, and slowly lift up your trunk. Alternative position: Push feet against the wall, and support your upper back with your hands as you lift your trunk.

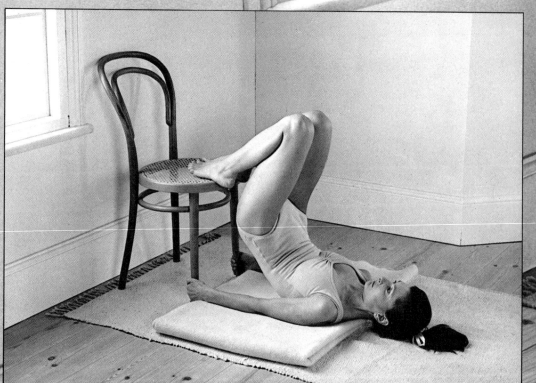

3 Hold the chair legs as you come up on to your shoulders. Your feet should be firm and steady on the chair, taking some of your body weight. Tuck shoulder blades under to increase support of back and spine. Stretch up through your spine, and hold position for several minutes. Alternative position: Push your feet against the wall, and support your upper back with your hands as you come onto your shoulders.

To come down, uncurl your spine slowly. Bring your hips down last. Breathe out slowly and continuously as you come down. Observe effects of this stretch on your body before continuing another move. In the "less-stretch" positions, the weight of your hips is taken by your legs.

·UPSIDE DOWN·
MORE STRETCH

If you find the basic position on pages 42 and 43 easy to do, you can achieve a greater stretch by bringing your legs down over your head. Only go as far as you can while still stretching your back up. Use a chair or a stool if the stretch is too hard. It is important to feel relaxed and happy in the position. Never force yourself so far that you become uncomfortable. Use a thick blanket under your shoulders to protect your neck.

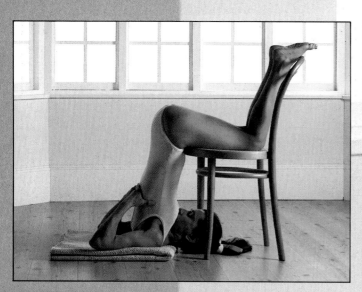

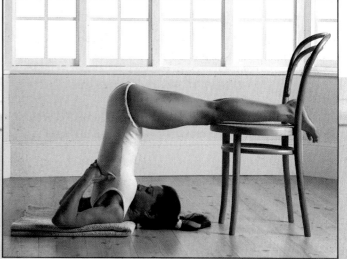

1 Place a chair behind you. Lie flat on your back. Bend your knees and raise them, first over your waist, then over your head, as shown in steps 1, 2 and 3 on page 42. Rest your knees on the seat of the chair. Support your back with your hands. Keep chin tucked into sternum. Wait until you are comfortable in this position before trying the next.

2 Stretch your legs straight out along the chair so they are at a right angle to your trunk. (It helps if you can get someone to move the chair back for you.) With the chair still supporting the weight of your legs, continue to lift your spine while supporting your back with your hands.

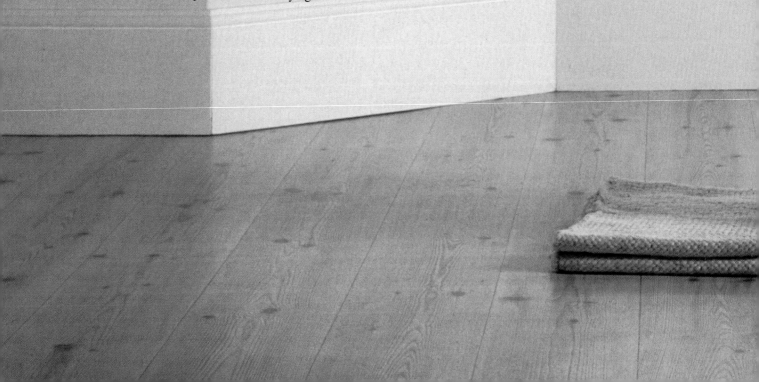

3 After some practice, if you find the stretch comfortable using the chair, try stretching your legs out lower. At first use a pile of books or a low stool as support for your feet. Keep your knees well-stretched, and support your back with your hands. If you can hold this for a few minutes without curving your back and collapsing, take your feet down to the floor. Stretch your arms toward your feet.

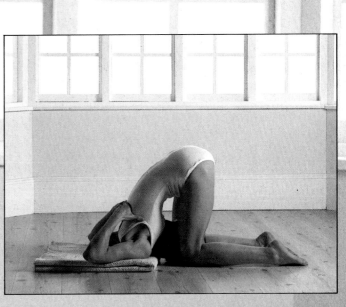

4 For the fullest stretch in your upper back and neck, use your hands to support your back. Bend your knees, and place them on either side of your ears.

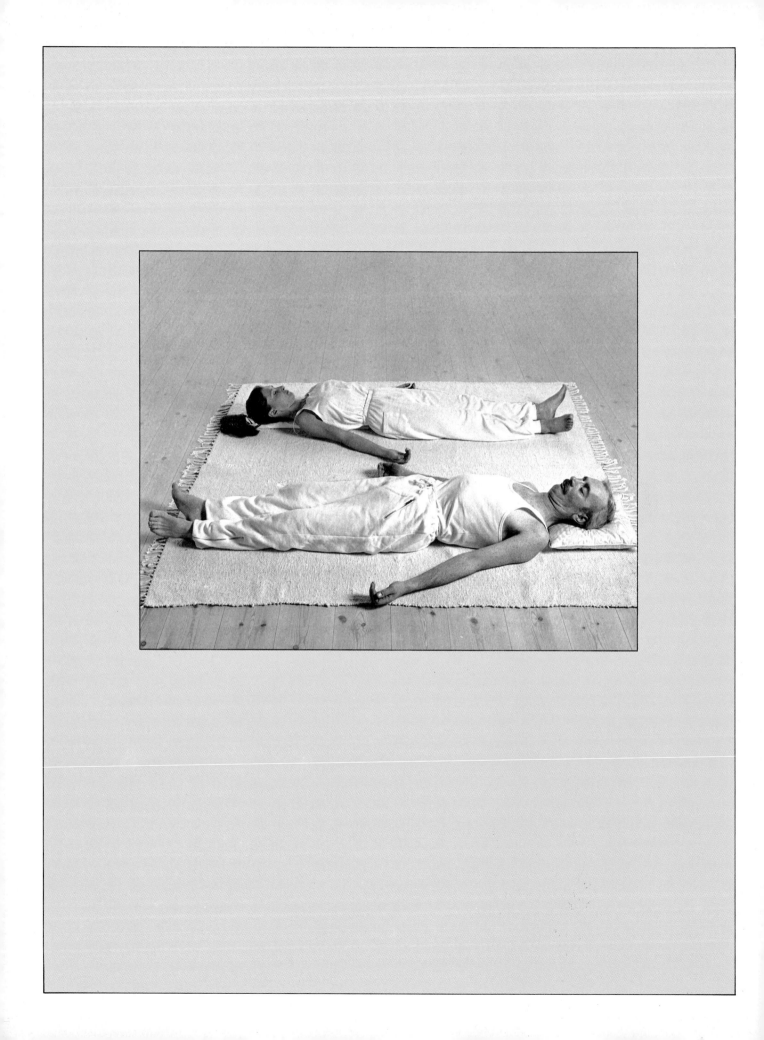

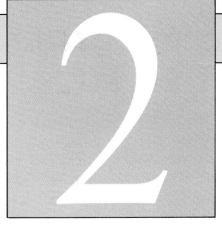

·RELAX·

The stress of daily living depletes energy and may lock tensions in your body. Relaxation enables you to follow activity with periods of rest and tranquility. It is not an escape from the pressures of modern life but a chance to replenish spent energies. Far from being a luxury, it's an essential part of living.

For some people, an absorbing hobby or sport provides a valuable form of recreation and a welcome antidote to the pressures of daily life. Yet, while sports and hobbies can be helpful and relaxing, they can also create new areas of tension. There are no substitutes for a brief daily period of total peace and quiet.

On a purely physical level, relaxation releases tension in the muscles. Your circulation improves, and your heart rate and blood pressure are regulated. But true relaxation is more than this. There is a release of tension in your body and a calming effect on your mind as the rhythms of your brain change. This isn't the same as going to sleep. When you begin to practice relaxation, you may fall asleep, but being asleep does not necessarily mean you are relaxed.

When you relax, you automatically breathe more slowly because your body needs less oxygen. This natural gentle rhythm can be a useful focus for your attention. The way you breathe is dictated by many things, including posture, tension and habit. As your body becomes strong and flexible through stretching and your posture improves, the way you breathe can change. At first, let your breathing improve naturally.

After a few months, when relaxation comes naturally and easily and your chest expands properly as you breathe in (see page 55), start to practice breathing slowly and more deeply. This increases your intake of air without using up unnecessary energy. Don't think of deep breathing as a discipline you impose on yourself. It is an extension of the relaxed state, achieved without straining. It should bring with it a feeling of refreshment and rejuvenation. If it feels difficult or strange when you first start, don't force it. Concentrate instead on improving your posture, stamina and flexibility in the stretches. Continue to practice relaxation until you feel ready to try again.

·HOW·TO·RELAX·

Learning to release muscular tension is fairly easy, but most people find it harder to unwind mentally. No matter how relaxed your body may feel, it is often hard to banish unwanted thoughts and worries and keep them from flooding into your mind. The relaxation techniques discussed here will help you relax mentally and physically. Do not be despondent if at first your mind continues to race; keep practicing, and you will find you are able to relax and unwind more each day.

The ideal time to practice relaxation is *after* you have completed a daily stretch program. Extending and flexing the spine and releasing tension in the joints and muscles will make you feel refreshed and able to let go. Another effect of stretching is to concentrate your attention on the movement of your body. As you focus on what you are doing, you will acquire a feeling of wholeness, a feeling that should stay with you as you lie down to rest at the end of the practice session.

How to lie down to relax is important. Your body must be evenly supported so you do not tilt to one side as you relax and thus set up a new pattern of tensions inhibiting deep relaxation. For this reason, it is unsuitable to lie curled up on one side or on your back with your head turned. The classic position for relaxation is shown in the photo opposite, while pages 52 and 53 suggest some suitable alternative positions for people who may find the basic one uncomfortable.

The basic position
The two stages of the classic position for relaxation are shown here. Start with your knees bent and your feet flat on the floor (see photo at right). Then extend your legs one at a time without arching your back (see photo above right).

Practicing relaxation
Choose a warm, quiet place away from bright light. Take the phone off the hook. Remove glasses or contact lenses. Spread a thick, soft blanket on the floor, and lie down on your back. Bend your knees, and place your feet flat on the floor close to your buttocks. Let the back of your waist drop toward the floor. Relax the strong muscles of your pelvis.

Without tensing your muscles, gently extend the curve at the back of your neck. Your chin will come down slightly, but your throat should stay relaxed. Let your eyes close.

As you breathe out, release tension in your shoulders by letting them drop down to the floor.

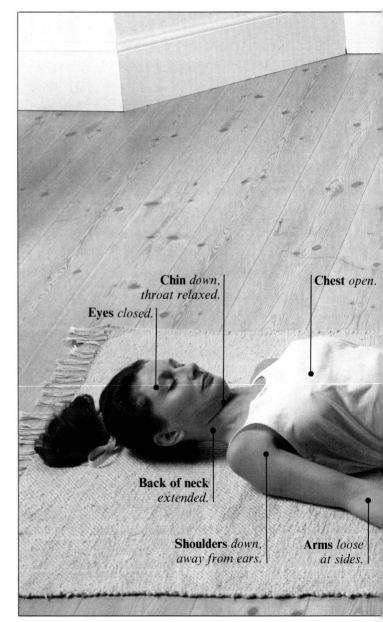

Chin *down, throat relaxed.*

Eyes *closed.*

Chest *open.*

Back of neck *extended.*

Shoulders *down, away from ears.*

Arms *loose at sides.*

Your arms will fall away from your body with the palms of your hands toward the ceiling. Your fingers will curl naturally. As your shoulders relax, your chest expands horizontally, and there is a feeling of space, which helps your breathing. Try not to let your chest cave in.

Extend your legs one by one, stretching from your hips to your heels. Let your feet fall apart naturally. As you breathe out, let the weight of your body sink into the floor. Continue to breathe gently, allowing the quiet and stillness to permeate your body. This takes time to achieve, so be patient.

Concentrate on your face. Let your muscles relax so the skin of your face feels smooth, especially across your forehead. Let your tongue rest behind your lower teeth. Relax the corners of your mouth, and keep your eyes closed. As your eyes become still, your brain begins to relax.

As you breathe, pause for a second at the end of each out-breath. Sink your pelvis, spine, arms and the back of your head into the floor. This should seem like a natural extension of your breathing. Let go of any residual breath, then allow the in-breath to come of its own accord. At first you will breathe consciously, but after a time it will be automatic. The gentle rhythm of breathing brings deep relaxation. Even at the end of a hectic day you will feel refreshed and revitalized.

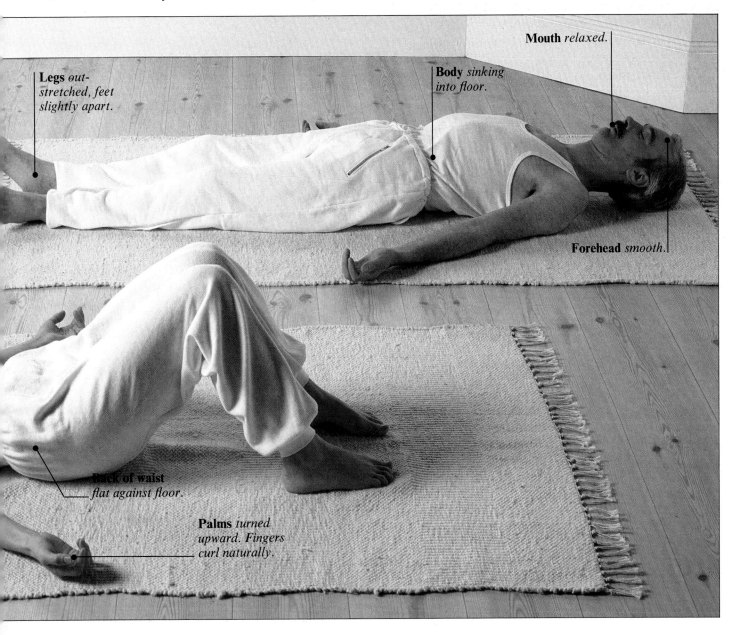

Legs *out-stretched, feet slightly apart.*

Body *sinking into floor.*

Mouth *relaxed.*

Forehead *smooth.*

Back of waist *flat against floor.*

Palms *turned upward. Fingers curl naturally.*

·ALTERNATIVE·POSITIONS·

If for some reason you find lying flat and still uncomfortable, then practice any of the alternative positions on these pages. The important thing is to practice relaxation every day after you finish the more dynamic stretches.

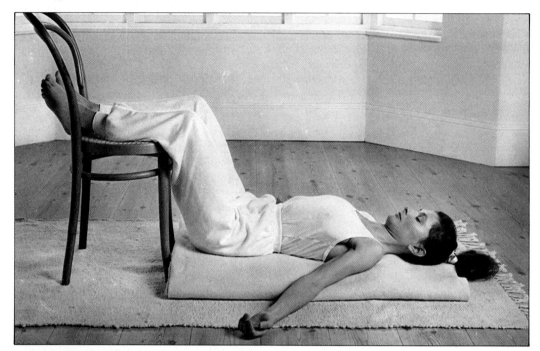

Easing swayback
If you have a swayback (see page 93) that arches up when you lie down, you will find it hard to relax lying flat. Instead raise your legs, and support your calves on the seat of a chair. (If you have only a slight swayback, a cushion or rolled blanket under your knees may be enough to ease the tension at the back of your waist.)

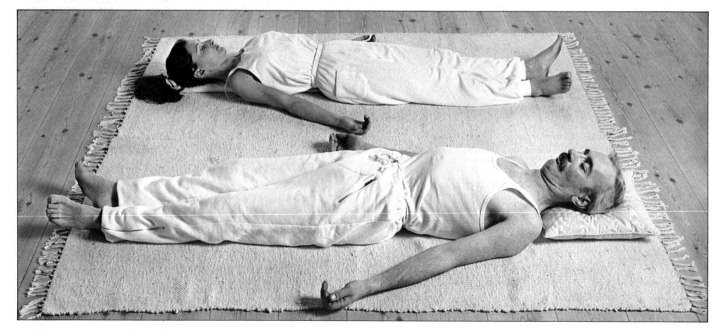

Easing stiff shoulders
If you find it difficult to relax your arms and shoulders, lie with your spine resting on a tightly rolled blanket. This will help to release tension in your shoulders and open your chest. The blanket should extend from the back of your hips to the back of your head. It must be narrow enough for your arms and shoulders to drop toward the floor.

Easing stiff neck and upper back
If your upper back is stiff and stooped, the basic relaxation position is not suitable. Your head will tilt back, the curve at the back of your neck will tighten and your chin will tip up too far. Allow your neck to extend freely by putting one or two pillows under your head. You should be able to relax your throat and jaw muscles.

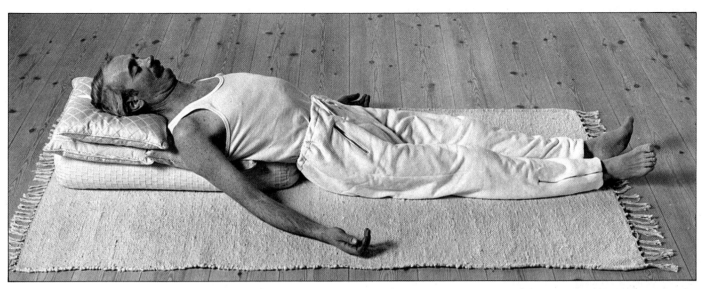

Easing breathing problems

Lying flat is not a good position for anyone with breathing problems. Instead use pillows to support your entire spine, from the back of your pelvis to your head. Your arms should be free to extend away from your shoulders. Stretch them gently to release stiffness before you close your eyes.

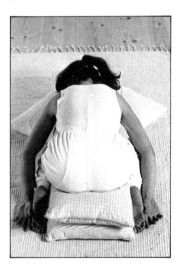

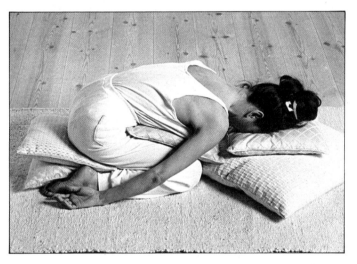

Kneeling forward

If you do not feel at ease lying flat on your back, this position is ideal. Keeping your spine straight, kneel on a blanket. Stretch forward onto pillows, and let your trunk relax. Support your buttocks on your heels or on small pillows.

Sitting forward

Try this position if you find your mind stays active when you relax. Sit with your legs together and straight. Put some pillows on top of them. Stretch out along the pillows, which should provide enough support to keep your spine from collapsing. The front of your body should feel extended, and you should be able to breathe easily. Do *not* use this position if you have back problems.

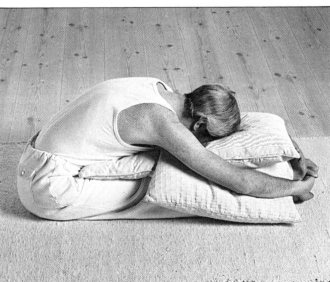

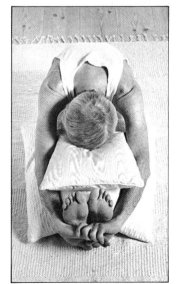

·DEEP·BREATHING·

Most of the time you probably pay little attention to the way you breathe. Perhaps you suddenly become aware of it during or after physical exercise – if you are breathing rhythmically while swimming, for instance, or if you are out of breath after running. You may not realize how your emotions also influence your breathing – you may sigh when depressed or hold your breath for a moment in anger. The reverse is also true – by concentrating on your breathing you can use it to influence your emotions.

Effective deep breathing
It takes patient practice to understand how to deepen your breathing while remaining quiet and relaxed. Generally you take a deep breath because you need more oxygen, and you use additional muscles to help you breathe. But this is stressful. Think of a runner gasping at the end of a race, forcing the muscles of his neck and shoulders to lift his ribcage. Avoid straining and struggling with the muscles of the upper chest. Instead try to increase the efficiency of your diaphragm and the efficiency of the muscles that lie between your ribs.

Learning to breathe correctly
Lifelong habits, such as faulty posture, affect the way you breathe. The long muscle fibers at the back of your diaphragm extend down your lumbar spine. Your diaphragm works more effectively when your spine is strong and flexible and correctly aligned. A body toned by stretching exercises will be more fit for deep breathing than one that is weak and poorly aligned. Other factors play a part in forming breathing patterns – tight clothes, such as belts or bras, restrict the movement of your body and can alter the way you breathe.

Be sure you know how to breathe correctly *before* you start to practice deep breathing. This is as important as making sure your individual posture is correct before you start to stretch and exercise. If you lie flat with your hands on your abdomen, ribcage and chest, as shown in the photos on the opposite page, you will be able to feel the correct movements. At first, rest between each stage, and breathe normally for a while. Eventually you will feel the entire movement in the course of one deep in-breath. After that you will no longer need to use your hands as a guide to the correct movement.

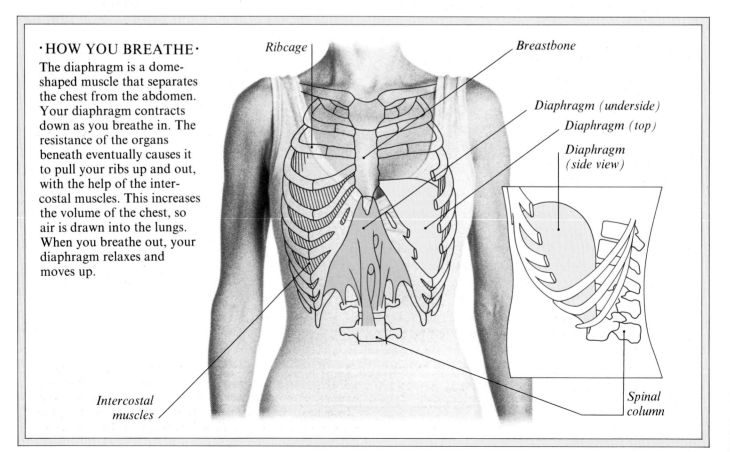

·HOW YOU BREATHE·
The diaphragm is a dome-shaped muscle that separates the chest from the abdomen. Your diaphragm contracts down as you breathe in. The resistance of the organs beneath eventually causes it to pull your ribs up and out, with the help of the inter-costal muscles. This increases the volume of the chest, so air is drawn into the lungs. When you breathe out, your diaphragm relaxes and moves up.

Ribcage

Breastbone

Diaphragm (underside)

Diaphragm (top)

Diaphragm (side view)

Intercostal muscles

Spinal column

If you find it impossible to breathe correctly this way, stop trying to do any deep breathing for a while. Concentrate on the stretches and the relaxation. As you practice the stretches, your body will gradually become flexible, and you will tone your abdominal muscles. This will help correct faulty breathing patterns. The lift from the lower abdomen and expansion of the chest in the "wide and strong" positions (see pages 22 to 25) are particularly effective.

Practicing deep breathing
When you first start to practice deep breathing, it is best if you lie down in one of the relaxation positions as described on pages 50 to 53. Wait a few minutes until your body feels relaxed, and you feel the quiet, even rhythm of your breath. Start by breathing out, beyond the point where you would normally stop. Continue to release tension. Let go of as much of the remaining air in your lungs as you can, although this may seem very little at first. As you come to the end of the breath, pause for about a second so you feel completely still, then breathe in slowly and deeply. Keep your face, tongue and throat relaxed as you do this. Focus your attention on the movement of your breath. Feel your ribcage gradually expand, with the lower ribs opening first. When your upper ribs move a little at the end of the breath, be sure to keep your neck and shoulders still. Pause for a second, and feel the back of your body resting on the floor.

Breathing in should not make you increase the curve at the back of your waist or neck. Your spine should still be relaxed and supple, not hard or rigid. Breathe out slowly as before.

To begin with, it can be difficult to learn the right techniques. If you breathe too slowly, you may feel suffocated. At first try one breath out and in, followed by a few ordinary breaths. If you feel like yawning, you need to breathe in a little more freely, and increase the volume of breath more quickly. Each breath should be smooth and steady with no jerks so you breathe in and out at the same rate from beginning to end. When you feel comfortable doing this, practice continuous deep breathing, establishing a regular pattern of in-breaths and out-breaths of even length. When you finish, be still for a while before you get up. You should feel relaxed and fresh afterward.

Breathing correctly

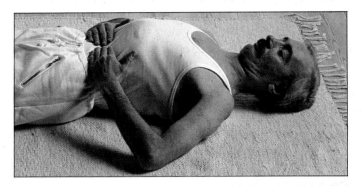

1 Lie on your back on the floor, and put the palms of your hands on your abdomen, with fingers pointing inward. Your middle fingers should be by your navel. Breathe deeply, and feel the movement of your abdominal wall beneath your hands. As you begin to breathe in, your abdomen should not push outward or upward against your hands but should stay flat. Any movement should be slightly down, away from thumbs and index fingers.

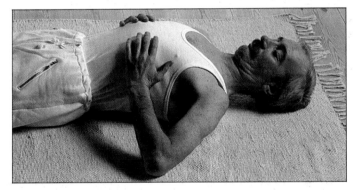

2 As you come to the middle of the deep in-breath, put your hands on your lower ribs with fingers pointing inward. Feel your lower ribs opening out sideways, moving your hands apart.

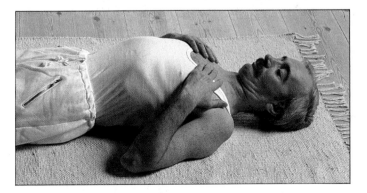

3 Continue breathing deeply. Put your hands high on your upper chest with fingers pointing inward and thumbs and index fingers just below your collarbones. Because the ribs here are fixed, movement will be less, but at the end of the deep in-breath, you should be able to feel a movement upward, toward your hands.

·ALTERNATIVE·POSITIONS·

When you have mastered deep breathing while lying relaxed on the ground, try sitting upright. An upright position, with the spine aligned correctly in its four curves (see page 92), is the ideal one. This is because when you lie down, your diaphragm is slightly displaced, so your in-breath is less efficient. Sitting up straight without tension requires strength and flexibility, and most people find it hard to hold the correct position for long in the beginning. It is difficult to combine sitting up and breathing deeply and rhythmically with keeping your neck and shoulders completely relaxed and your spine stretching upward. Trying to impose a pattern of deep breathing on a stiff, tense body makes you feel restless and disturbed. Deep, even breathing should come as a natural extension of a calm mind and a relaxed body.

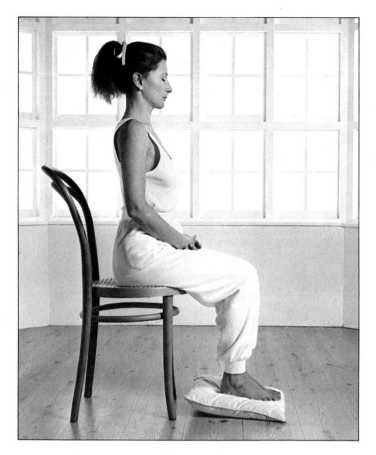

Sitting on a chair
The easiest way to sit with your spine aligned in its natural curves is to sit on a hard-backed chair with feet and thighs comfortably supported and your back straight. Do not lean against the chair back, but sit up tall and relax your shoulders. If the chair is too low sit on a pillow. If it is too high, put a pillow or a book under your feet.

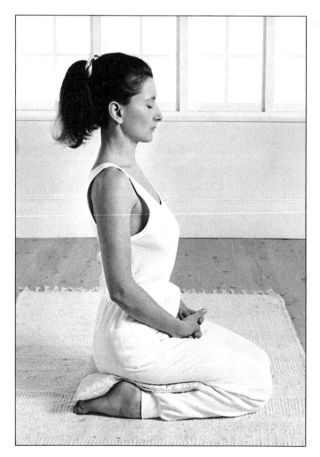

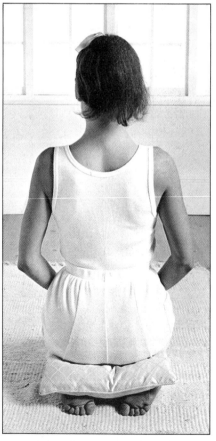

Sitting on your heels
This is a good position in which to keep your back erect and your shoulders relaxed. But if you sit like this for long, you may get pins and needles in your feet. Try sitting with a folded blanket or pillow on your heels. Be sure feet and knees are straight, and the weight is evenly distributed.

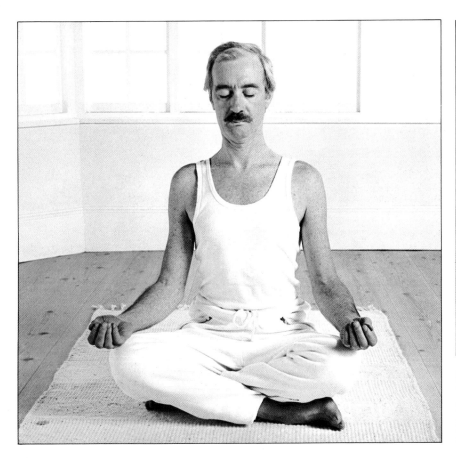

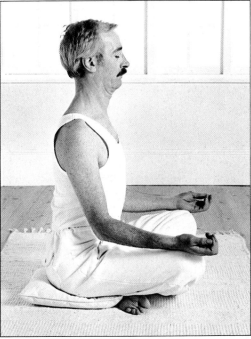

Sitting cross-legged on pillows
The position of your legs tends to push you backward a little, so sit on as many pillows as it takes to raise your trunk comfortably. Keep your feet on the floor.

Sitting cross-legged
If you have flexible hip joints, sit on the floor with your legs crossed. Your weight should be a little to the front of your buttock bones. You may find it hard to keep shoulders relaxed with your hands on your knees as shown above. It depends on the length of your arms and the stretch and flexibility of your spine. You can put your hands in your lap where you feel most comfortable (see photo at right). If you use the cross-legged position, alternate the way you cross your legs.

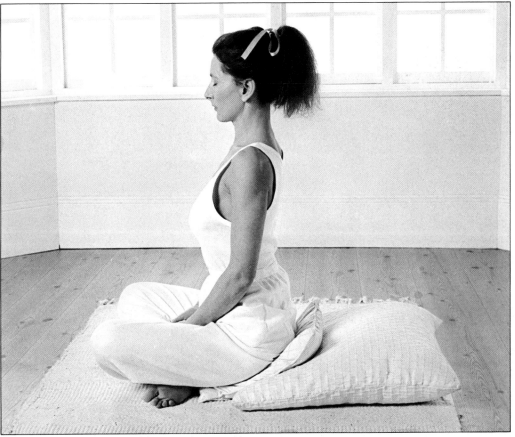

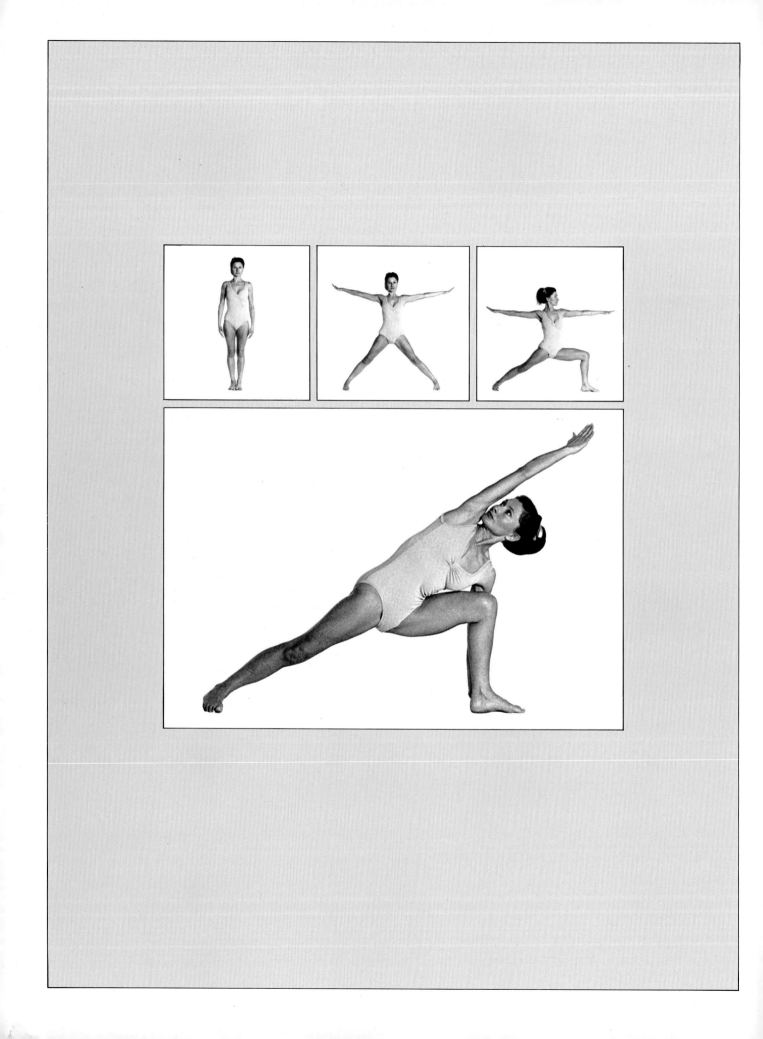

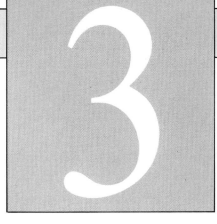

·STRETCH·PROGRAMS·

Methods of exercising that promise instant transformation are suspect and dangerous. Change must take place gradually: you can't force your body to loosen up overnight. If you want to tone it up and make it fit and more supple, regular practice is essential. The ideal is a short daily session, but it's better to exercise a few times each week than to go all out for the occasional extended practice. It is also safer and more effective to practice for 20 minutes each day than to exert yourself frantically each week for a couple of hours.

Your daily practice must be planned and developed with care; over a period of weeks and months your body will change. Because everybody is different, five programs have been devised; each is designed to last about 20 minutes. The beginners' program is ideal if you have never done any stretching before. The basic program should be eventually within the range of most people. The program for very stiff or elderly exercisers can be a practice in itself or serve as an introduction to the beginners' program. The program for more-supple exercisers is designed for those who have practiced the basic program for many months and who feel the need to extend more. The final program is for people who are more experienced, who have practiced for at least 1 year and who would like to give more time to daily practice.

You'll get the most out of the daily programs if you're already familiar with Chapter One; or you'll need to keep referring to the detailed instructions for each stretch. If you can't do the upside-down stretches at the end of each program, finish by repeating the appropriate back-to-the-center position. As you progress to more-demanding programs, give more time to difficult positions. Relax into them gently, without straining. Stretch and relaxation go together; as you increase the stretch, spend longer in the upside-down position. Take more time relaxing at the end of the practice, including doing some deep-breathing exercises while lying down.

The last two programs on pages 70 to 73 are slightly different. They are relaxation programs that last about 1 hour. Practice them once a month, on a day when you can give yourself a complete rest and stay at home quietly.

·BEGINNERS·

In this program you learn how to feel the correct movement of the spine. Practice it for a few months before moving on to the basic program. If you are stiffer than average, you may find the program on pages 64 and 65 more suitable for the first few weeks. Begin by holding the stretches for a few seconds only. Increase the time as your body gets used to regular practice.

1 **Straight**
See page 17.

Place weight evenly on both feet. Keep back long, shoulders relaxed. Stand straight, stretch up through spine. Hold for 1 minute.

2 **Sideways**
See page 20.

Spread feet 36 inches apart. Keep knees straight and arms out to side. Keep spine extended and chest open. Stretch sideways only, not forward. Do not try to go down too far. Hold for 30 seconds on each side.

3 **Wide and strong**
See page 24.

Spread feet 54 inches apart. Keep arms out to side. Stretch arms straight up above head. Keep back long, knees straight. Hold for a few seconds, then stand up. Repeat twice. Increase to 30 seconds.

4 **Back to the center**
See page 28.

Kneel straight, and sit on heels. Stretch arms up over head. Hold for 1 minute. Bend forward, keeping hips straight, and arms by your side. Hold for 1 minute.

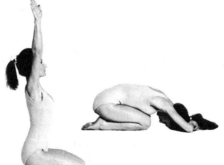

5 **Forward**
See page 32.

Sit up tall, with legs straight out in front of you. Hold for 30 seconds. Bend forward from hips, keeping back straight, and catch toes with hands. Keep shoulders relaxed. Hold for 30 seconds.
Use a belt if you cannot reach your toes easily, or do a forward stretch shown on page 64.

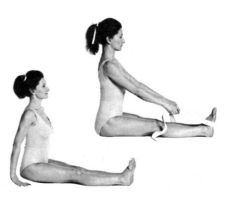

6 Twist

See page 36.

Place chair so it cannot slip. Face chair, and put one foot on the seat, with thigh parallel to the floor. Twist around, and stretch up. Open your chest, and relax your shoulders. Hold for 30 seconds on each side.

7 Backward

See page 40.

Lie on your stomach, with arms at your sides. Lift legs and shoulders off floor. Begin leg lift by tightening muscles under buttocks. Lengthen spine, open chest and stretch back of neck. Do not take feet higher than head. Hold for a few seconds, and repeat twice. Increase to 30 seconds.

8 Upside down

See pages 42, 43 and 46.

Lie on blanket. Press palms against floor, and raise legs over waist with knees bent. Swing knees over head, and straighten legs. Keep head straight, neck long and elbows in. Stretch up toward feet, lifting from upper back. Hold for 3 minutes. Put legs back on chair, keeping back long and stretching up. Rest knees on chair seat. Hold for 2 minutes.

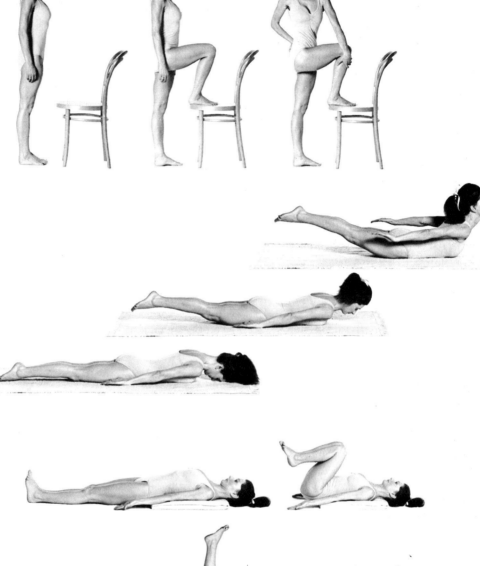

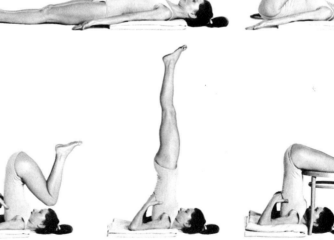

9 Relax

See pages 50 to 53.

Lie with head, spine, arms and hands well-supported on pillows. Keep neck long. Stay in position for at least 5 minutes. If this is uncomfortable, try one of the other positions described on pages 50 to 53.

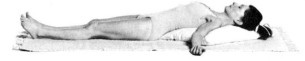

·BASIC·

This program shows you how to put together, in sequence, the basic stretches. Initially practice the "beginners" program on pages 60 and 61, but eventually the stretches here should be within the range of most people. Even if you are very flexible, practice this program for several months before moving on to a more advanced one.

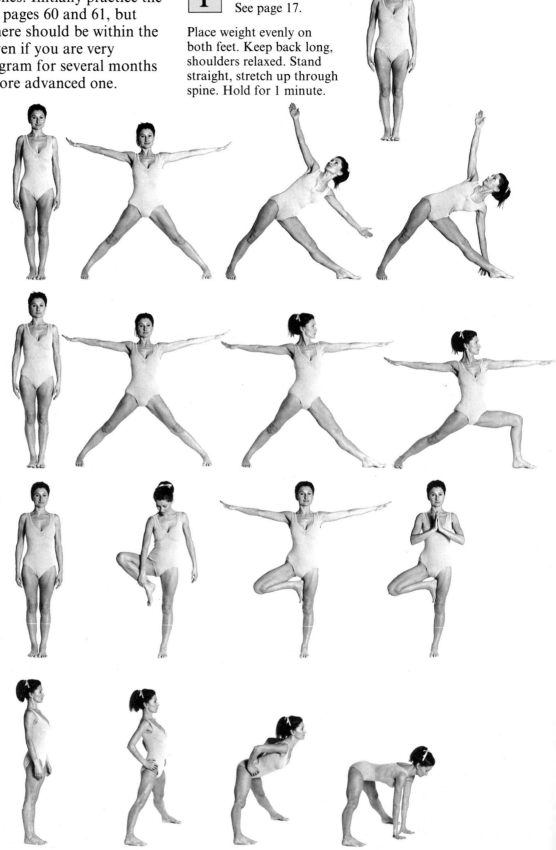

 1 Straight
See page 17.

Place weight evenly on both feet. Keep back long, shoulders relaxed. Stand straight, stretch up through spine. Hold for 1 minute.

2 Sideways
See pages 18 and 19.

Spread feet 36 inches apart. Keep knees straight, and arms out to side. Keep spine extended and chest open. Stretch sideways only, not forward. Hold for 30 seconds on each side.

3 Wide and strong
See pages 22 and 23.

Spread feet 54 inches apart, with arms out to side. Make thigh of bent leg parallel with floor, and keep other leg straight. Hold for 30 seconds on each side.

4 Back to the center
See pages 26 and 27.

Press one foot into other thigh. Keep standing leg straight and foot pointing forward. Extend lower back, and keep the abdominal muscles firm. Relax shoulders. Press hands evenly. Hold for 30 seconds on each side.

5 Forward
See pages 30 and 31.

Spread legs very wide apart, about 60 inches. Place hands on hips. Bend forward, keeping hips and head in line. Lengthen back. Hold with head up for 1 minute *or* hold for 30 seconds with head up 30 seconds with head down.

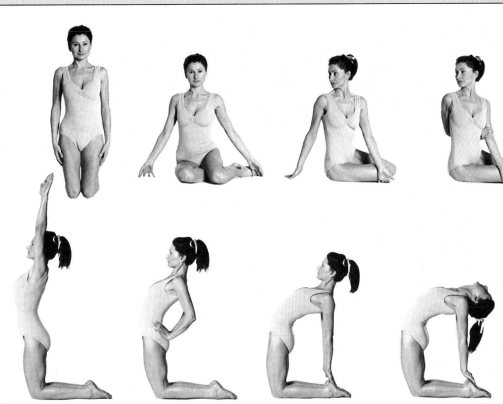

6 Twist

See pages 34 and 35.

Kneel with weight evenly on your knees. Sit back on heels, with legs folded behind you. Stretch up as you turn. Relax shoulders, and open chest. Grasp arm behind back. Hold for 30 seconds on each side.

7 Backward

See pages 38 and 39.

Kneel on knees and feet straight. Push forward with hips. Lift spine, open chest and catch heels with hands. Extend neck, taking head back. Hold up to 30 seconds.

8 Upside down

See pages 42, 43 and 46.

Lie on blanket. Press palms against floor. Raise legs over waist, with knees bent. Swing knees over head, and straighten legs. Keep head straight, neck long and elbows in. Stretch up toward feet. Lift from upper back. Hold for 3 minutes.

Take legs back onto chair, keeping back long and stretching up. Have feet together, knees straight, and legs resting on seat. Hold for 1 minute.

9 Relax

See pages 50 and 51.

Lie with spine long, and weight falling evenly on hips and shoulders. Keep head straight. Hold for 1 minute with knees bent. Hold for at least 4 minutes with legs straight.

·LESS·SUPPLE·

You may want to practice this program for a few weeks before starting the program for beginners on pages 60 and 61, but it was also designed as a daily practice for people who are particularly stiff. Gradually increase the length of time you hold each position. Do not hold your breath as you stretch. Release gently into the positions without strain.

 Straight
See page 17.

Place weight evenly on both feet. Keep back long, shoulders relaxed. Stand straight, stretch up through spine. Hold for 1 minute.

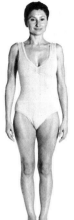

 Sideways
See page 20.

Spread feet 36 inches apart. Keep arches lifted with knees straight. Stretch out as you reach sideways to chair. Look up, and relax neck and shoulders. Hold for a few seconds. Repeat twice on each side.

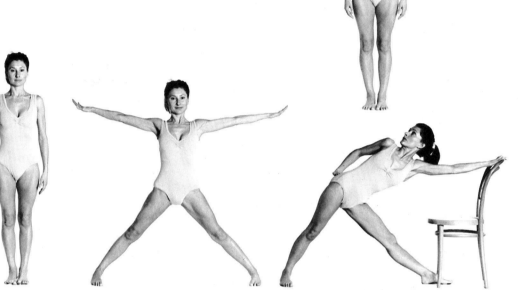

 Wide and strong
See page 24.

Spread feet wide apart. Keep legs straight and toes forward. Release shoulders as you stretch wide. Hold for a few seconds, then stand straight. Repeat twice.

 Back to the center
See page 28.

Lie flat on your back with weight evenly distributed. Relax your hips as you bend one leg. Keep other leg straight on floor and knee tight. Hold for 1 minute on each side.

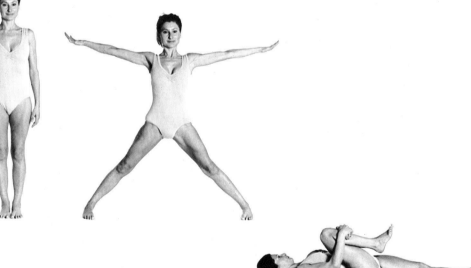

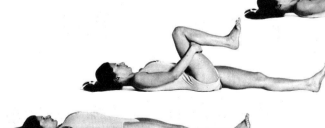

5 Forward

See page 32.

Stand straight, with arms over head. Bend from hips, as you stretch toward the chair. Keep feet slightly apart and toes pointing forward, knees straight, not hyperextended. Lengthen back, and relax shoulders. Hold for 30 seconds.

6 Twist

See page 36.

Sit tall, keeping hips straight. Stretch up as you turn head in line with hips. Relax your shoulders. Hold for a few seconds, then repeat twice on each side.

7 Backward

See page 40.

Put chair so it cannot slip. Kneel straight, and push hips forward. Lift up as you bend back. Hold for a few seconds. Repeat position twice.

8 Upside down

See pages 44 and 45.

Place a blanket under shoulders and back. Hold the chair so it cannot slip. Keep head straight. Press feet against chair seat, and roll up from upper back. Tighten muscles under buttocks. Tuck in shoulder blades. Hold for up to 2 minutes.

9 Relax

See pages 50 and 53.

Lie with head, spine, arms and hands well-supported on pillows. Keep neck long. Stay in position for at least 5 minutes. If this is not comfortable, try one of the other positions on pages 50 to 53.

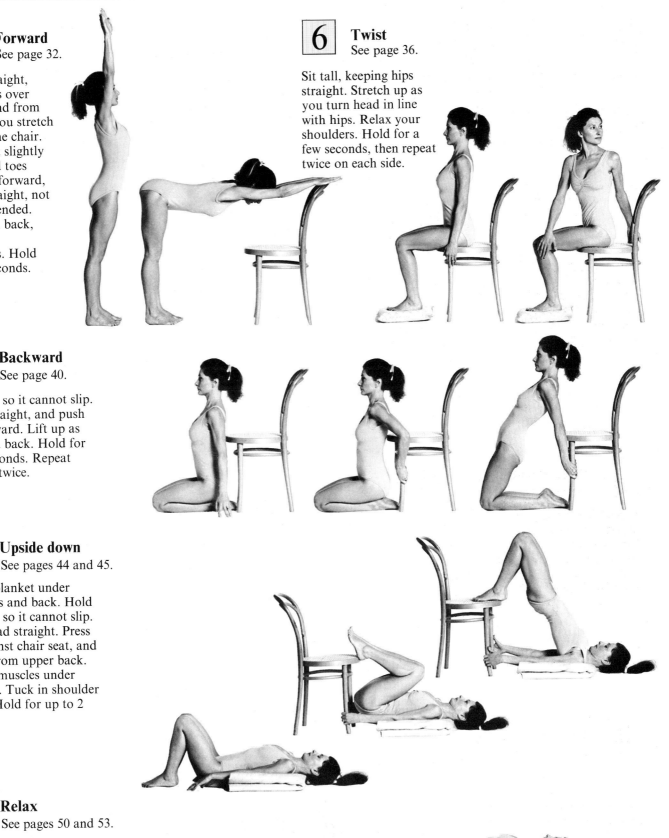

·MORE·SUPPLE·

If you are strong and supple, you may feel after some months of regular practice that you need to stretch more in the stretches than the basic program allows. If you want to, practice this program twice a week while doing the basic program on the other days.

 Straight
See page 17.

Place weight evenly on both feet. Keep back long and shoulders relaxed. Stand straight, and stretch up through spine. Hold for 1 minute.

2 Sideways
See page 21.

Spread feet 54 inches apart, knees straight, arms out to side. Keep spine extended, chest open. Press outside of back foot against floor, make front thigh parallel with floor. Stretch diagonally to side, look up. Hold for 20 seconds each side.

3 Wide and strong
See page 25.

Spread feet 54 inches apart, and stretch arms up above head. Turn entire body. Lower hips, make front thigh parallel with floor. Keep back leg straight. Open chest, stretch up. Hold for 20 seconds each side.

4 Back to the center
See pages 26 and 27.

Press one foot into other thigh. Keep standing leg straight and foot pointing forward. Make back long, as you relax shoulders. Press hands evenly. Hold for 30 seconds on each side.

5 Forward
See pages 30 and 31.

Spread legs very wide apart, about 60 inches. Bend forward, keeping hips and head in line. Lengthen your back. Drop head right down, with hands between feet and elbows bent. Hold for 1 minute, allowing spine to lengthen gradually on each out-breath.

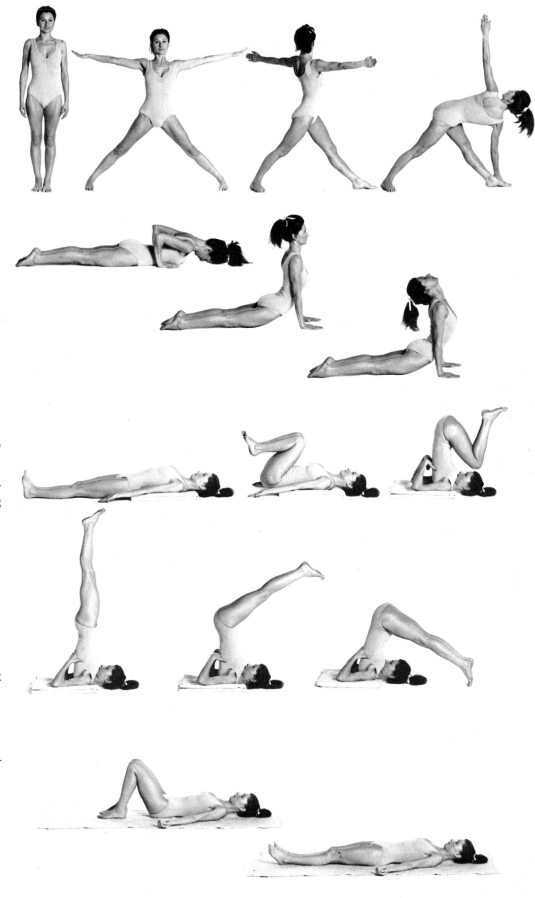

6 **Twist**
See page 37.

Spread feet 36 inches apart, and keep legs straight. Rotate from hips, and extend right arm over left foot. Make back long and open chest. Stretch top arm up, and turn head. Hold for 20 seconds each side.

7 **Backward**
See page 41.

Lie on front with body straight. Lengthen spine. Lift up with arms straight and chest open. Extend neck, and take head back. Put weight on hands and tops of feet only. Hold for 20 seconds, repeat twice.

8 **Upside down**
See pages 42, 43, 46 and 47.

Lie on blanket. Press palms against floor. Raise legs over waist with knees bent. Swing knees over head, then straighten legs. Keep head straight, neck long, and elbows in. Stretch up toward feet as you lift from upper back. Hold for 5 minutes.

Place legs back on chair, pile of books or down to floor. Keep back long, and stretch up. With feet together, keep knees straight and arms supporting upper back. Hold for 3 minutes.

9 **Relax**
See pages 50 and 51.

Lie with spine long, weight falling evenly on hips and shoulders. Keep head straight. Hold for 1 minute with knees bent and 4 minutes with legs straight. Introduce some deep breathing. See pages 54 and 55.

·ADVANCED·

This program is suitable for people who have practiced our stretches for a year or more, who have a good understanding of their bodies and who would like to give more time to their practice. Allowing for extra relaxation time, this program takes about half an hour.

 Straight
See page 17.

Place weight evenly on both feet. Keep back long and shoulders relaxed. Standing straight, stretch up through spine. Hold for 1 minute.

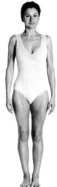

 Sideways
See page 21.

Spread feet 54 inches apart. Keep knees straight and arms out to side. Keep spine extended and chest open. Press outside of back foot against floor. Make front thigh parallel with floor. Stretch diagonally to the side and look up. Hold for 20 seconds on each side.

 Wide and strong
See page 25.

Spread feet 54 inches apart. Keep knees straight and arms up over head. Turn entire body. Lower hips, and make front thigh parallel with floor. Keep back straight. Open chest, and stretch up. Hold for up to 20 seconds.

Straighten standing leg, and lift back leg, keeping knee straight. Extend ankle. Stretch out arms. Back foot and hands should be level. Hold for 20 seconds. Repeat sequence on other side.

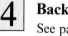 **Back to the center**
See page 29.

Sit on floor with legs straight. Spread legs very wide. Bend knees, and bring soles of feet together. Let knees drop toward floor, and lift spine. Hold for 1 minute.

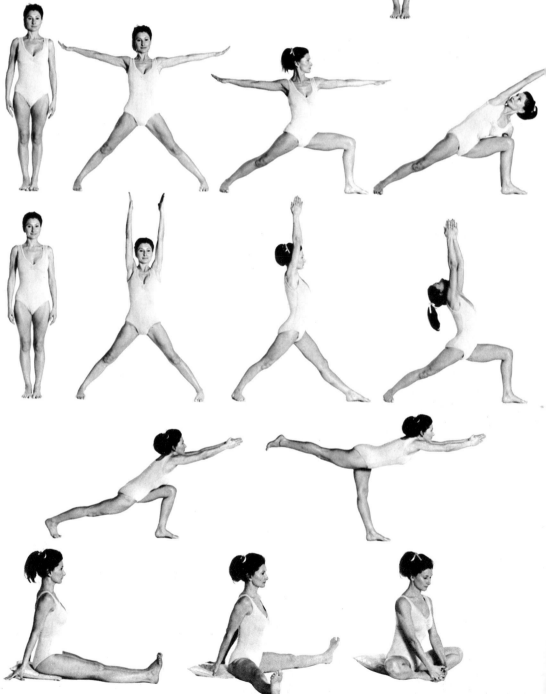

Forward

See page 33.
Stand with feet together.
Raise arms above head.
Bend forward, and place
fingers on floor next to toes.
Keep knees straight. Stretch
forward with head up. Hold
for 1 minute. Bend down
from hips, and grasp ankles
with hands. *Do not* pull at
feet. Hold for 2 minutes.
(Work up to 5 minutes once
a week).

 Twist

See page 37.

Sit with legs straight. Bend
right leg. Twist around to
right. Place left arm around
right knee, and catch hands
behind back. Hold for 20
seconds each side. Repeat.

 Backward

See page 41.

Lie on floor, and stretch out
with arms above head. Bend
knees. Bring heels close to
hips. Raise hips, and lift
trunk. Tighten muscles
under buttocks. Lengthen
spine, and open chest. Arch
back, and curve chest. Hold
for 10 seconds.

 Upside down

See pages 42, 43 and 47.

Make body vertical. Keep
head straight, neck long, and
elbows in. Hold for at least
7 minutes.
   Take legs back down to
floor. Hold position with
knees straight for 3 minutes.
Keep chin tucked into chest.
Bend knees close to head.
Hold for 2 minutes.

 Relax

See pages 50 and 51.

Lie with spine long and
weight falling evenly on hips
and shoulders. Keep head
straight. Hold for 10
minutes. Do deep breathing
at least three times a week,
once a week in a sitting
position. See pages 54 to 57.

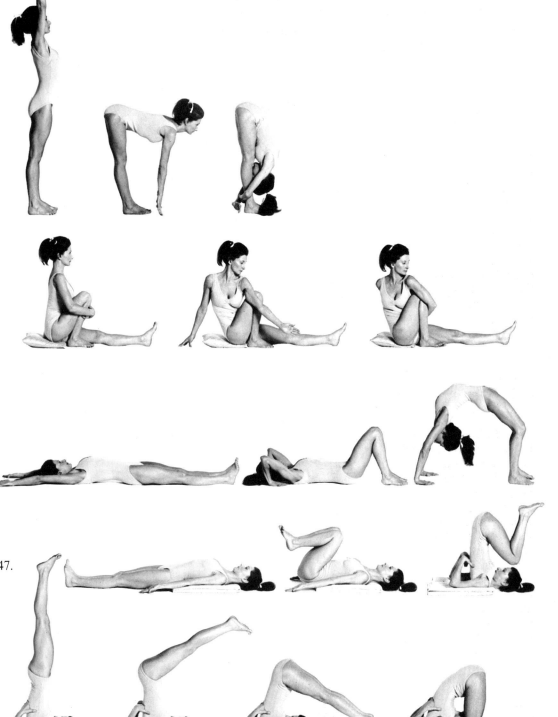

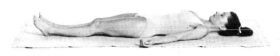

·RELAX·
LESS STRETCH

If you practice the "less-supple" or "beginners" daily program, you might like to try this more extended relaxation program occasionally, perhaps once a month. The aim is to relax fully, not force or overextend yourself. Breathe slowly and deeply as you hold the positions to release muscular tension as you stretch.

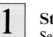

1 Straight
See page 17.

Place weight evenly on both feet. Keep back long and shoulders relaxed. Standing straight, stretch up through spine. Hold for 2 minutes.

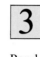

2 Up
See page 32.

Spread feet about 12 inches apart. Keep them parallel. Keep knees straight but not hyperextended. Stretch arms up above head. Breathe in as you lift arms, and breathe out as you stretch tall. Extend lower back, and keep the abdominal muscles firm. Hold for 2 minutes. Breathe normally. Repeat twice.

3 Forward
See page 32.

Bend from hips. Keep feet slightly apart, toes pointing forward and knees straight. Lengthen back, relax shoulders and open chest. Hold for 30 seconds.

4 Forward
See page 32.

Spread legs very wide apart, about 60 inches. Breathe out, and bend forward with hips and head in line. Lengthen back, and relax shoulders. Take head and hands down to chair seat. Hold for 30 seconds.

5 Upside down
See pages 44 and 45.

Place blanket under shoulders and back. Hold chair so it cannot slip. Keeping head straight, press feet against chair seat. Lift from upper back. Hold up to 2 minutes.

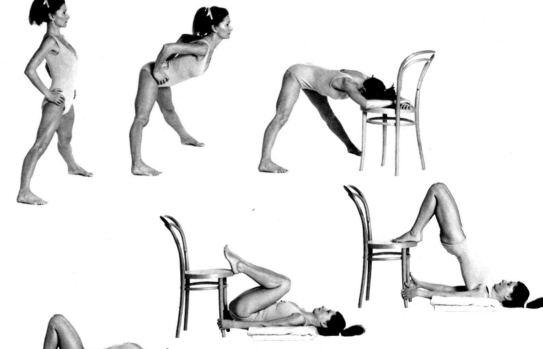

6 Flat
See page 42.

Lie on floor. Stretch out, with arms above head. Lengthen spine, particularly waist and neck. Hold for 2 minutes.

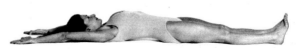

7 Upside down
See page 46.

Place blanket under shoulders and back. Lie flat on floor with knees bent, heels close to buttocks. Lift from upper back onto tops of shoulders. Place legs back on chair, keeping back long and stretching up. Rest knees on chair, and take arms down. Hold for up to 2 minutes.

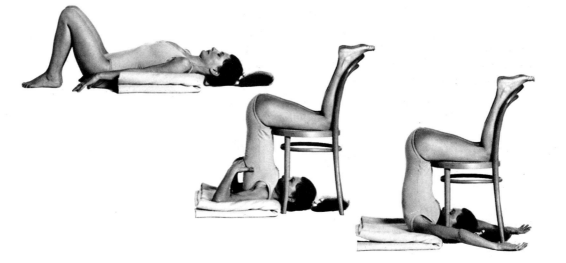

8 Flat
See page 42.

Lie on floor. Stretch out with arms above head. Lengthen spine, particularly waist and neck. Hold for 2 minutes.

9 Back to the center
See page 28.

Lie flat on your back with weight evenly distributed. Relax hips as you bend one leg. Keep other leg straight on floor, with knee tight. Hold for 1 minute on each side.

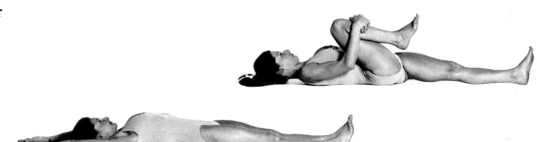

10 Back to the center
See page 28.

Kneel straight, and sit on heels. Stretch arms up over head. Bend forward, with hips straight and hold for 1 minute.

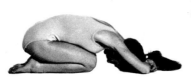

11 Back to the center
See page 28.

Breathe in as you come up from previous position. Stretch up. Breathe out, relax shoulders and stretch arms right up. Hold for 1 minute.

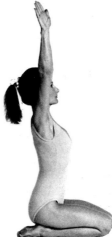

12 Relax
See pages 50 to 53.

Lie with head, spine, arms and hands well-supported on pillows. Stay in position for at least 10 minutes, then practice deep breathing for 5 minutes. Finish by relaxing for 5 minutes more.

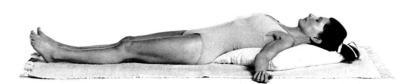

·RELAX·
MORE STRETCH

You can do this relaxation program if you regularly practice the programs for the more supple or experienced. It offers you the opportunity, once a month, to spend more time in the positions than in everyday practice. Breathe deeply as you relax in the stretches.

 Straight
See page 17.

Place weight evenly on both feet. Keep back long, shoulders relaxed. Stand straight, stretch up through spine. Hold for 2 minutes.

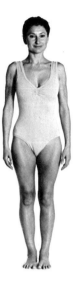

 Up
See page 32.

Stand with feet together. Keep legs straight and stretch arms over head. Breathe in as you take arms up, and breathe out as you stretch tall. Hold for 2 minutes, breathing normally. Repeat twice.

 Forward
See page 33.

Bend forward from hips. Keep knees straight. Stretch forward with head up. Hold for 1 minute. Bend from hips, relax trunk and let head drop as neck relaxes. Hold elbows, and stretch arms away from shoulders. Hold for 2 minutes.

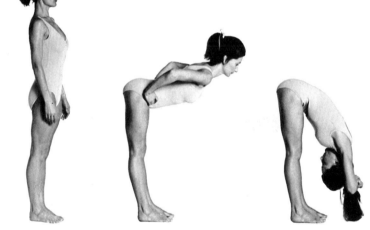

 Forward
See pages 30 and 31.

Spread legs very wide apart, about 60 inches. Bend forward with hips and head in line. Lengthen back. Drop head down, with hands between feet and elbows bent. Hold for 1 minute.

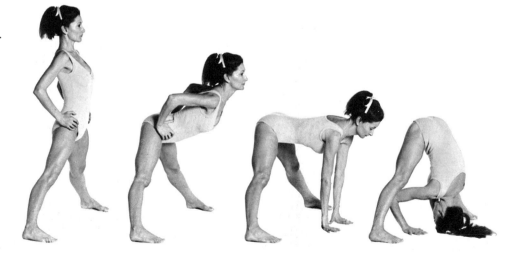

5 Upside down

See pages 42, 43, 46 and 47

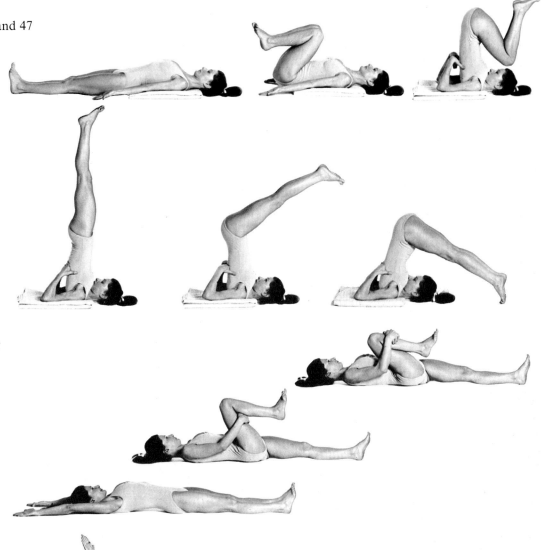

Lie on blanket. Press palms against floor, and raise legs over waist with knees bent. Swing knees over head, and straighten legs. Keep head straight with neck long and elbows in. Stretch up toward feet, and lift from upper back. Hold for at least 5 minutes. Experienced students can hold for 10 minutes. Place legs back on chair, pile of books or on floor. Keep back long, and stretch up. Keep feet together, with knees straight. Hold for up to 5 minutes. Experienced students can hold longer.

6 Back to the center

See page 28.

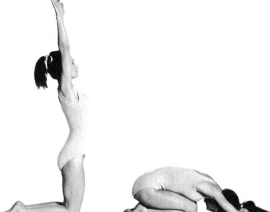

Lie on back, with weight evenly distributed. Relax hips as you bend one leg. Keep other leg straight on floor with knee tight. Hold for 1 minute on each side.

7 Back to the center

See page 28.

Kneel up, and stretch arms up over head. Hold for 1 minute. Bend forward with hips straight and arms out in front. Keeping hips down, lengthen back. Hold for 1 minute.

8 Relax

See pages 50 and 51.

Lie with spine long and weight falling evenly on hips and shoulders. Keep head straight. Stay in this position for 10 minutes, then practice deep breathing for 5 minutes. Finish by relaxing for 5 more minutes.

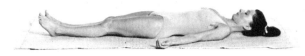

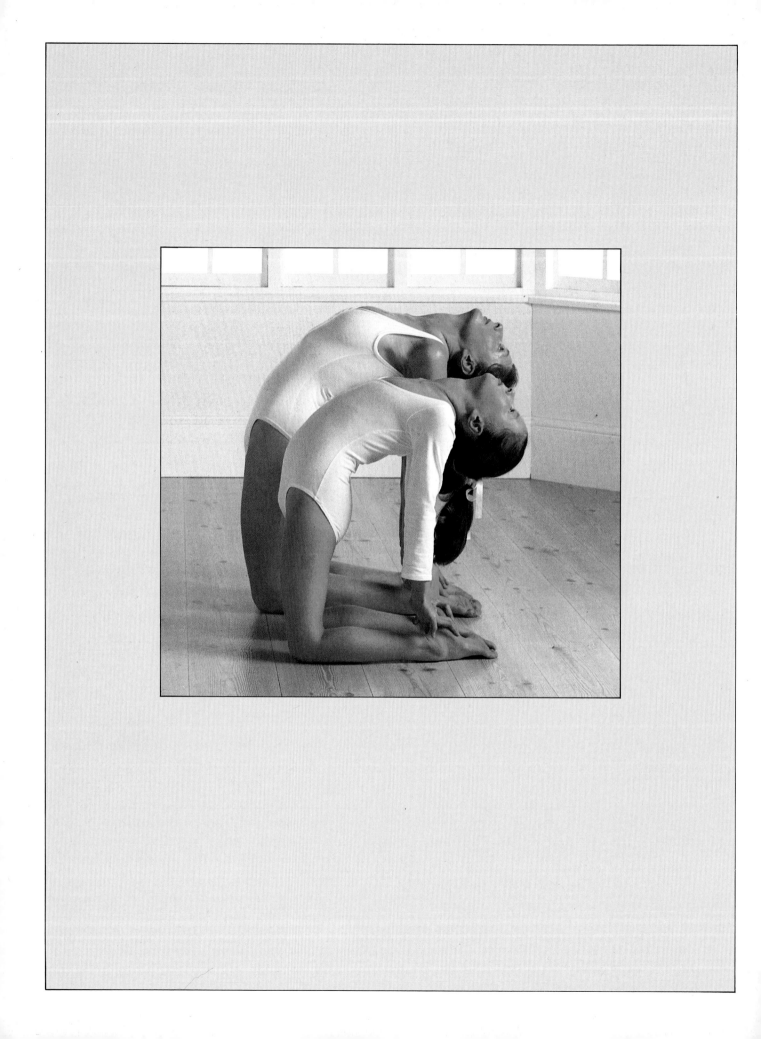

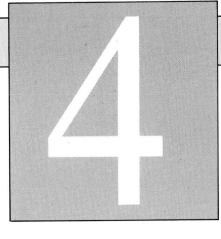

·STRETCH·TOGETHER·

Daily practice on your own is important because you need to concentrate without distraction. But occasionally – perhaps once a week – stretching with friends or family is fun, especially with children.

When you stretch in a group, it's crucial to know how to help each other properly. Before trying to help family or friends, make sure you have a good understanding of the spine (see pages 92 and 93) and basic stretches. Refer to the instructions in Chapter One for any stretch you try. Follow instructions carefully, then help each other. The instructions in this chapter are directed at the *helper*.

It's very difficult to judge what's happening to your spine when you start to stretch. You can correct the front of your body by looking at yourself in a mirror, but focusing your awareness on the *back* of your body needs more skill. This is where another pair of eyes helps. Take turns using a pole or broom handle to align each other's spines. Information on pages 76 and 77 explains how the pole should touch the back; this applies to all the stretches where the pole is used in this chapter. The touch of the pole brings the exerciser's awareness to the back of the body. If the spine collapses and shortens, it will push against the pole.

It's important to lie down and relax after practicing with other people. Take turns reading the instructions from Chapter Two. At the same time make sure your partner is lying straight.

Children don't have the concentration and stamina of adults, so don't be too serious about the way they move. Encourage them to feel good about their own posture, to think tall when standing or sitting and not to slouch in chairs. Use the pole the same way as for adults but not for too long. Adjust them quickly, or they'll get bored. They have more energy than adults and like to move more quickly from one position to the next. Never force them because their muscles and ligaments are weaker than an adult's. Let them stretch freely and naturally to keep their bodies mobile. It's good for children to relax for a few minutes afterward because they learn to appreciate a calm, quiet atmosphere. Although they enjoy relaxing with adults, don't expect them to stay quiet for as long – they don't have the patience.

·STRAIGHT·

Even people who feel they stand quite straight will find it helpful to have their posture checked occasionally with a pole. In a good standing position, there should be a little gap between the pole and the back of your partner's body at the waist and back of the neck.

Checking correct posture See page 17.

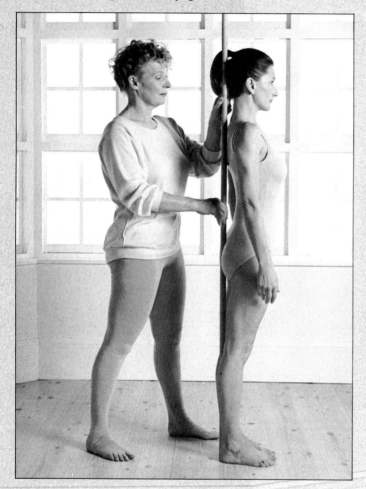

Let your partner find her natural position on her own as she stands up and stretches straight. Place the pole vertically behind her, so its base touches the back of her heels. In the correct position, the back of her head and her sacrum touch the pole, which also just brushes the back of her chest.

Identifying a swayback

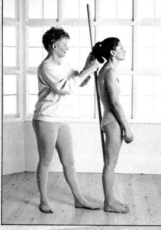

If your partner has a swayback, her upper spine will be very stiff and rounded. It will push the pole backward out of line. Tight back muscles will push her chin forward. For more about this problem, see the information about posture on pages 92 to 95.

Overcorrecting a swayback

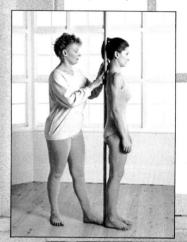

In trying to overcorrect a swayback, your partner may drag down her lower back and completely flatten her waist so there is no gap between the pole and the back of her waist. This is called a *flat back*. For more about this problem see pages 92 to 95.

Make sure *neck is long and head is straight.*

Drop *shoulders.*

Helping a child See page 17. Children sometimes slouch or droop, letting their heads hang down. After a while this can spoil their spinal alignment. Encourage your child to stand straight. Use a pole as you would to check an adult (photo opposite).

Let *hands relax.*

Keep *legs straight.*

Check *feet are parallel.*

·SIDEWAYS·

When helping a partner to stretch sideways, line up a pole on her spine *before* she starts to stretch to the side. This is shown on page 76. As she moves into the stretch, realign the pole so it lies along her spine in line with her feet. You'll be able to see at once if she goes out of line, and you'll realize how important the "less-stretch" positions are in achieving correct movement.

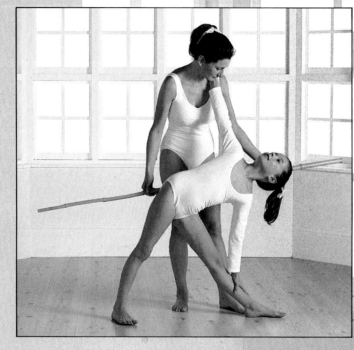

Helping a child See page 20. Encourage your child to stretch sideways, using a pole for guidance. Help her open her chest and stretch her top hand up. Don't make her hold the position for long, or she may become restless and lose interest in stretching.

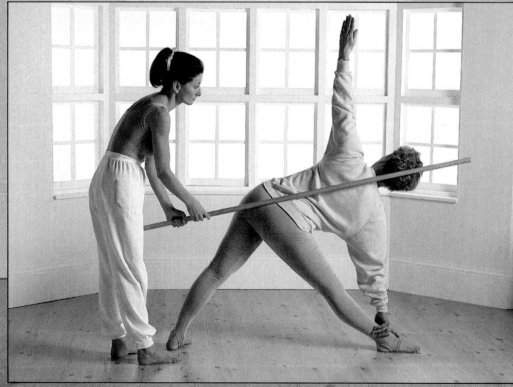

Basic and less stretch
See pages 18 to 20.
Hold a pole against your partner's tailbone. Follow the line of her feet. As she moves sideways, don't let the pole swing backward or forward. It should touch her sacrum and the back of her head, leaving only a small gap at the back of her waist and the back of her neck.

Make sure *outside of foot stays on floor.*

More stretch See page 21.

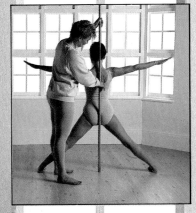

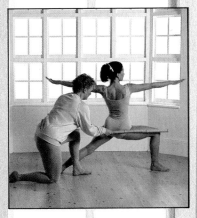

1 Hold a pole vertically behind your partner while she stretches tall. It should come down the middle of her body.

2 Hold the pole horizontal, and make sure your partner's thigh is parallel with the floor before she stretches any farther.

3 In the final stretch, keep the pole in line with your partner's feet so it touches the back of her heel, her sacrum, the back of her head and her upper hand.

Have *thigh parallel with floor.*

Keep *knee straight.*

Make *shin vertical.*

·WIDE & STRONG·

Although all the wide-and-strong positions can be done with a partner, help is especially useful with the balancing stretches. By offering a steadying hand, you can help your partner to concentrate on feeling the correct movement in the spine.

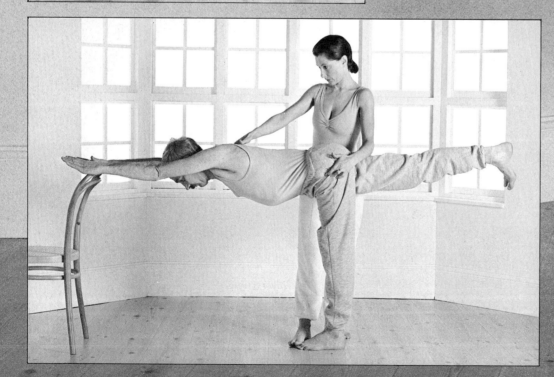

More stretch See page 25. Hold a pole vertically so your partner touches it with the bottom of his spine and the base of his skull. At first he should keep his hands on his hips and concentrate on feeling the correct stretch in his spine as he bends his front knee. Only after he can make a right angle at the knee should he move his arms above his head.

Lift *back leg up with knee straight.*

More stretch See page 25. Adults find this stretch difficult because stiffness in hips and shoulders and the fear of falling make it hard to stretch the spine fully while balancing on one leg. Get your partner to press his hands against the top of a chair. Help him keep his hips level by extending the hip of his standing leg. Check his alignment at the same time. His outer hip should be in line with his outer ankle, and his shoulders should be at the same level as his hips. He should stretch horizontally from his pelvis.

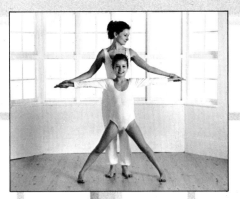

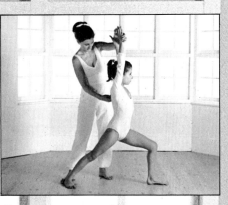

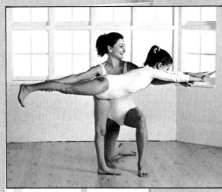

Helping a child See page 25.

1 As the child jumps her feet wide and spreads her arms, tell her to stretch into her fingertips. Make sure her arms are high enough.

2 As she breathes out and turns her front leg, help the child raise her arms over her head. When she bends her knee, let her find her own level for her hips.

3 Let the child move quickly into the final position without forcing the stretch. She will probably need a minimum of guidance. Make sure her body is horizontal, with her feet the same height as her hands.

Keep *back of neck long.*

Stretch *hands forward.*

Make *standing leg straight and strong.*

4 Children need encouragement to stay and stretch in the position for a few seconds. Doing the stretches together can provide the right motivation as well as being fun.

· BACK · TO · THE · CENTER ·

Applying gentle pressure to the thighs helps your partner stretch in these positions. (Never press directly against the knee joints because this can cause injury.) Your partner should not feel pain; you should merely help him or her to relax into the stretch. When helping children, don't use any pressure. Children can help adults, however, as long as they are careful and gentle.

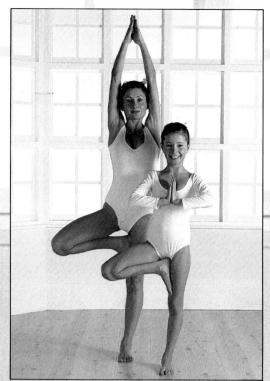

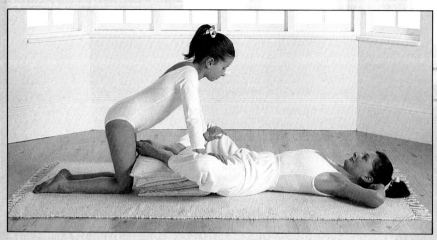

Hip stretch See page 106.
Be sure your partner is lying comfortably, with feet supported on pillows. Kneel down, and apply gentle pressure to her thighs. Rotate them outward and press on both thighs evenly. If your partner is very stiff, use more pillows. Make sure her feet aren't too near her hips. This stretch is an easier alternative to the "more-stretch" position. See page 29.

Basic stretch See pages 26 and 27.
Balance is a challenge to children and adults, so enjoy doing this stretch together. Try to concentrate and hold the position for as long as you can. Because adults have stronger leg and spinal muscles, they can move their arms above their head if they want an extra stretch. A child would find this hard.

Less stretch See page 28.
A child who is light can safely stretch over an adult in this position, as long as the child's feet remain on the floor. The adult benefits because the extra pressure applied keeps her buttocks down on her heels. She can then extend her spine and move forward more easily. Caution: Two adults should *not* help each other this way.

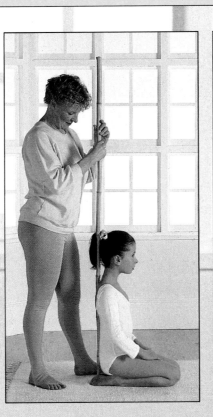

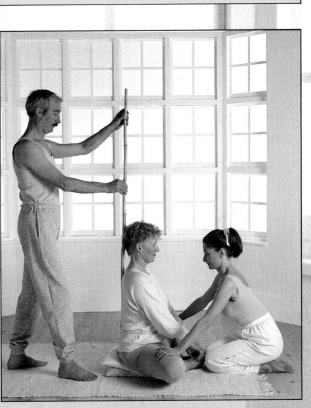

Less stretch See page 28. When your partner is sitting on her heels, hold a pole vertically against her back and see if she is stretching properly. Make sure her hips and feet are evenly placed and her pelvis is not tilted. Take away the pole so she is able to bend forward.

More stretch See page 29. Help your partner by gently extending her hips outward. Use only minimum pressure needed to encourage muscles to relax. Put your hands on her thighs, not on her knees. You can also help by using a pole.

Child *should keep back of neck long.*

Let *child's weight help your buttocks go down.*

Relax *shoulders and arms.*

·FORWARD·

Many people find movement from the hips is difficult in forward stretches because tight back thigh muscles (hamstrings) limit the rotation of the pelvis. This places extra strain on the lumbar spine. By using a pole for guidance, you help your partner understand the correct movement more easily and quickly.

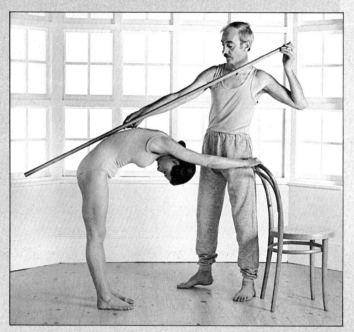

Less stretch See page 32. Place a pole behind your partner as she bends forward to touch a chair. She may curve her back as she bends and push the pole away from her sacrum and head (photo at left).

In the correct stretch, your partner's spine should be parallel with the floor (photo below), with the pole horizontal. For this to happen, the backs of her thighs must extend. This allows her pelvis to rotate forward and her lower spine to stretch out from her hips. Her legs should stay straight and vertical.

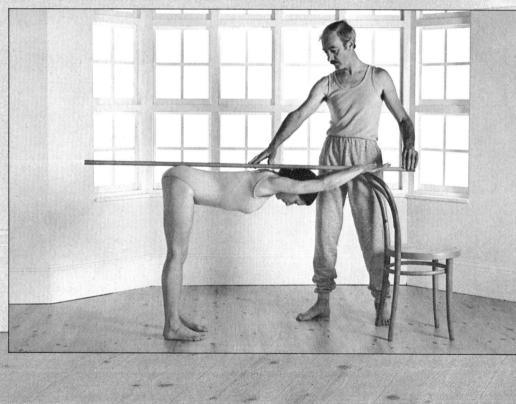

Roll *small stick forward along pole.*

Less stretch See page 32. Your partner can intensify the forward stretch of her spine. She can hold a small stick and push it along the big pole, with arms extended. She should keep her legs firm but may have her feet together or wide apart, as she prefers.

Lengthen *spine to go forward.*

Keep *hips directly above feet.*

Make sure *feet are parallel.*

·TWIST·

Help your partner feel the correct stretch in the twisting movements by using a pole for guidance. Other ways to increase his or her stretch are shown below. Choose the ones that seem appropriate. Make sure your partner is comfortable and not overstretching.

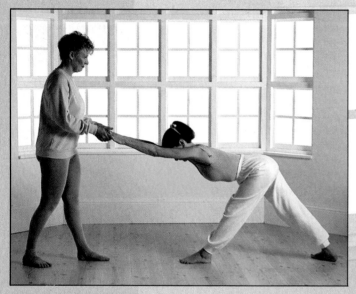

Extending forward See page 37.
Help your partner extend her spine, as she prepares to turn, by gently stretching her forward. Hold her hands high enough for her to move her lower back in.

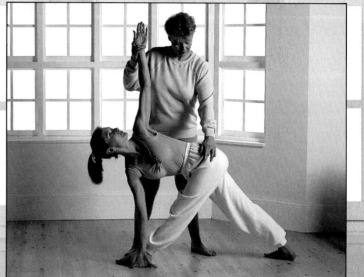

Extending the arm See page 37.
While your partner twists, hold her upper hand, and gently extend her arm up. This will help her turn her upper spine. Your hand on her hip will assist balance.

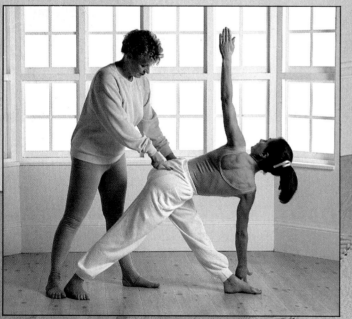

Extending hips See page 37.
As your partner turns to the left, gently extend her left hip backward to help her twist more effectively. Her lower back should move in.

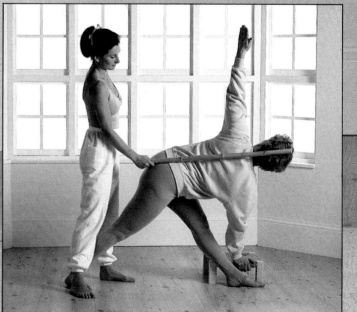

Using the pole See page 37.
Hold a pole behind your partner to help her feel the correct stretch. If she finds it difficult to turn properly, let her rest her hand on a stool instead of the floor.

Feel *back of head touch pole.*

Basic stretch See pages 34 and 35.
Rest the bottom of the pole on the floor so your partner's sacrum is touching it before he starts to twist. As he stretches up and twists around the pole, keep it absolutely straight.

Stretch *up spine as you twist.*

Feel *base of spine touch pole.*

·BACKWARD·

These stretches should extend the entire spine, not only the back of the waist. Helping someone in these movements makes it easier for him or her to stretch the spine while bending back. This is especially useful for someone who is stiff.

Less and basic stretch
See pages 38 to 40.
The stiffer your partner is, the more she will benefit from help. Pull her hips gently (photo at far right), encouraging her to stretch from her lower back. Or loop a belt around her bottom, near the tops of her thighs (photo at right). Don't hold her rigidly, but give her the support she needs to achieve a good stretch with confidence.

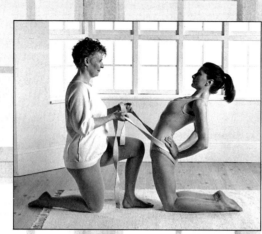 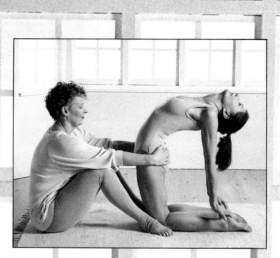

Less stretch See page 40.
It's good if two of you can help with this. First, ask your partner to lie on his front and hold the other helper's knees (or a piece of heavy furniture if there is only one helper). Grasp his heels, and gently pull back so as he bends backward, he can stretch against your resistance. Don't pull his feet up too high.

Stretch *back of neck.*

Lengthen *back of waist.*

Partner *should gently extend your leg.*

·UPSIDE·DOWN·
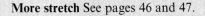

In these stretches, the upper back has to lift so there is no pressure on the neck. If your partner's head needs adjusting, she should come out of the position to straighten it.

Caution:
Never lift or pull people when they are upside down.

Basic stretch See pages 42 and 43.

More stretch See pages 46 and 47.

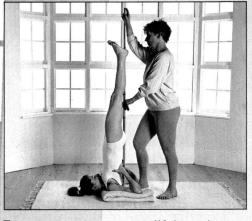

Encourage your partner to lift her spine against a pole. If she becomes red in the face, she should do the "less-stretch" pose.

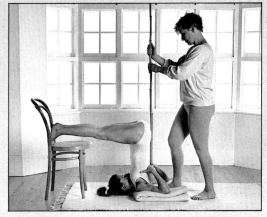

Your partner's spine should align with the pole. If her back collapses and pushes it away, she should lift her feet higher.

Basic stretch See pages 42 and 43.

Reach *forward with arms.*

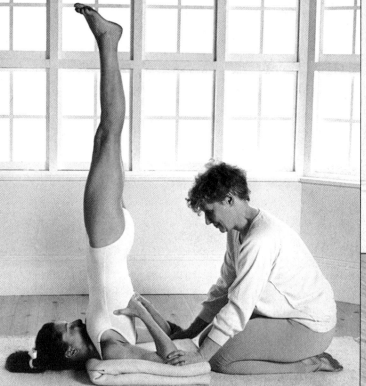

Help your partner get a good lift in her upper back by gently holding her elbows down. Keep them the same distance apart as her shoulders.

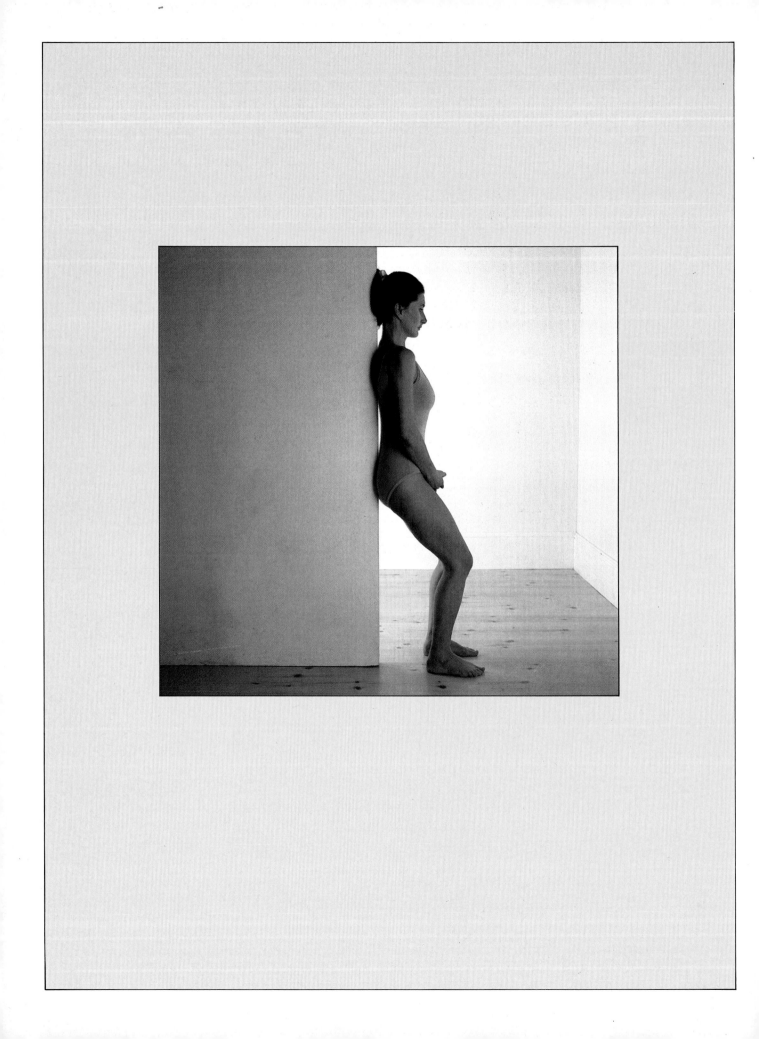

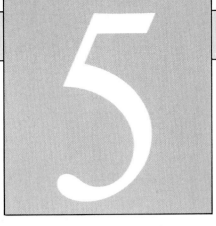

· RELIEVING · STIFFNESS ·

The perfect body is the exception, not the rule. The fact you're right- or left-handed causes uneven muscular development, so very few people stand really well or move as easily as they might be able to. If you do the same actions day after day, you develop certain patterns of movement, and inevitably you underuse your potential range. Your posture deteriorates; imperceptibly stiffness becomes habitual.

As long as you're healthy and carefree, you may remain unaware of the ill effects of poor posture. Most of the time you feel all right because your body is highly adaptive. It compensates with strong muscles taking over the work of weaker ones. As soon as you're tired, ill or emotionally upset, however, you become conscious of the strain. Stretching sensibly each way every day should help, but particular problems will benefit from the stretches in this chapter.

Part of the trouble stems from the way the human body has evolved. Originally designed for life on all fours, the human animal turned into a biped. In the process major skeletal changes took place. The pelvis tilted backward, and the new need to reach up and use hands caused the concave lumbar curve to develop. Eventually, the spine developed four curves (see page 92). A curved spine is stronger, more flexible and better able to withstand gravity than a straight one. Unfortunately, careless use of the body can upset the balance of the spinal curves. As a result, many people suffer from backache or related problems at some time. This chapter begins with the spine and goes on to discuss each part of the body. Information in this section helps you understand your posture and discover areas of stiffness. Learn to use your body correctly, and enjoy the freedom a greater range of movement brings.

The stretches in this chapter are intended to be done before your daily stretch program. Some are easy; others may seem a little more difficult, especially if a friend is checking you with a pole as you stretch. (See Chapter Four, pages 74 to 89.) Go slowly and use common sense when you try the stretches. If you have any doubts, consult your doctor before you start. Remember that relaxation and stretch go together. You will discover your tensions and areas of stiffness while relaxing and stretching, so treat relaxation as an essential part of relieving stiffness.

·SPINE·

The spine is an engineering masterpiece. It is flexible and stable at the same time. Similar to a ship's mast, the spinal column is inserted into the pelvic "deck" and rises up to the head. It supports the shoulder girdle in the same way as the mast supports the weight of the sails. Muscles and fibrous bands, called ligaments, hold it in place. This structure allows the body to stabilize itself as it moves.

What causes backache?
The spine's flexibility can be restricted by incorrect usage, which can cause several back problems. A sudden twist at an awkward angle or an excessive strain on one part of the spine can have a painful effect on the spinal column and muscles and ligaments. To farther complicate things the spinal cord runs through a channel along the spine, from the top of the neck to the lumbar region. Because of this, trouble with a vertebra can put pressure on part of the nervous system. Back problems can be a cause of pain in almost any part of the body.

Most backaches have no obvious causes – but poor posture contributes to back pain. If you stand tall, sit straight, lie on a firm bed, wear flat shoes and lift heavy objects by bending at the knees, you're doing what you can to protect your back. Information on the next 3 pages describes common postural faults and good stretches to correct them. On pages 96 and 97 is a program of stretches to ease backache. Information on pages 98 and 99 covers specific back problems, with suggestions for stretches to relieve them.

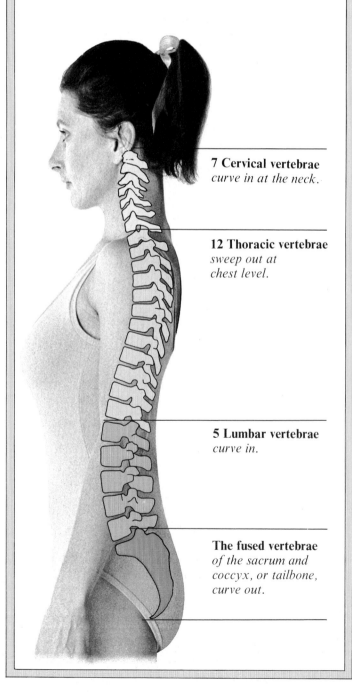

·THE SPINAL COLUMN·
The spine, or backbone, stretches from the bottom of the buttocks up to the base of the skull. It is made up of more than 30 bones, called *vertebrae*. The vertebrae are linked by fibrous ligaments and powerful muscles, which make the whole structure strong and flexible. The vertebrae also protect the spinal cord, which is the central channel of the nervous system.

7 Cervical vertebrae
curve in at the neck.

12 Thoracic vertebrae
sweep out at chest level.

5 Lumbar vertebrae
curve in.

The fused vertebrae
of the sacrum and coccyx, or tailbone, curve out.

Good posture

Stand against a wall or door, and look in a mirror. If you are standing tall, your spine will curve in at your neck and waist and out at your upper back and sacrum. There should be gaps between your body and the door at the back of your neck and the back of your waist *only*.

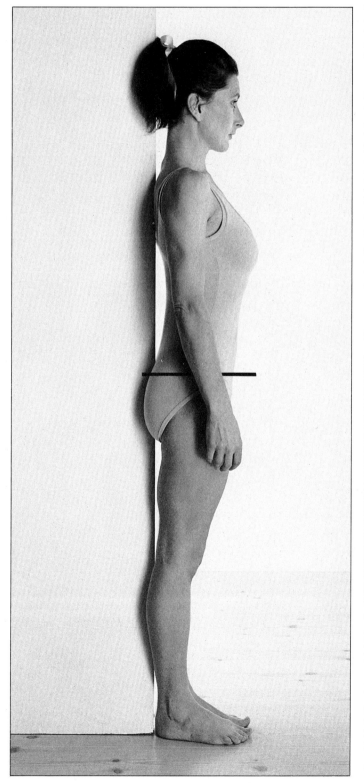

Identifying your back type

Every object has a center of gravity, with its weight evenly balanced around that center. In the human body, this center lies inside the upper part of the pelvis – a little higher in a man than a woman. When everything is correctly aligned, the curves of the spine are well-balanced, and the pelvis is horizontal (photo below left). Two common types of incorrect posture are shown below, and the black lines show the pelvis is no longer horizontal.

Checking your posture

Understanding often comes from seeing because habitually faulty posture *feels* correct. Look in a mirror at your spine from the side. Notice how you hold your shoulders and head, whether you push the back of your waist in deeply and notice if your abdomen sags. Be critical of yourself. If it's difficult to see properly in a mirror, ask someone else to check you (see pages 76 and 77), or try standing against the edge of a door with your heels touching it. The next page shows how to correct poor posture.

Swayback

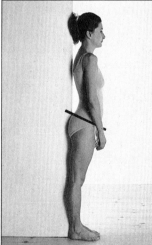

Flat back

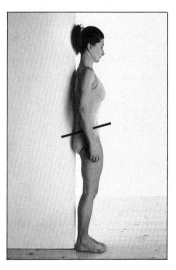

This defect is more common in women, often because high-heeled shoes pitch the body weight forward. Because the body weight is taken by the toes, if the spinal muscles are weak the pelvis tilts forward. The top part of the trunk sways back, causing an excessive curve at the waist.

A flat back is more common in men. The pelvis is tilted up at the front so there is hardly any lumbar curve. Rounded shoulders and a weak spine are part of this droopy look. It results in a rigid, more easily damaged spine and can cause breathing and digestive troubles.

·CORRECTING·POSTURE·

Poor posture can be corrected by strengthening back and abdominal muscles. It takes time before you feel the change in your body, but for a little effort you will be rewarded by good posture. It feels right, looks good and helps your entire body function better.

Start by thinking tall. Lift from your pelvis, tuck in your tailbone, extend your spine and drop your shoulders. Do the stretches that apply to you every day. Concentrate on feeling the changes in your muscles as you stretch. In time good posture will become second nature.

Stretch for a swayback
Rest your back against the edge of a door, with knees bent and feet 6 to 9 inches away from the door. There should be as little space as possible between the back of your waist and the door (photo at right). Relax the muscles in the hollow of your waist, and take a few deep breaths. Slowly straighten your knees, and slide your spine up the door. Tighten abdominal muscles to keep your back flat (photo at far right). You should feel your upper spine lift, while your waist stays long at the back. Hold for a few seconds, then gently bend your knees, and repeat two or three times.

Next try the stretch with your heels closer to the door. Avoid increasing the gap at your waist.

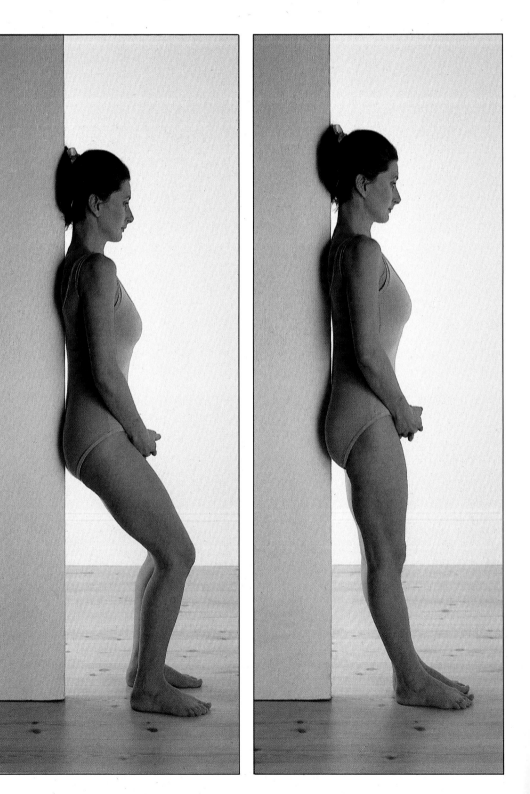

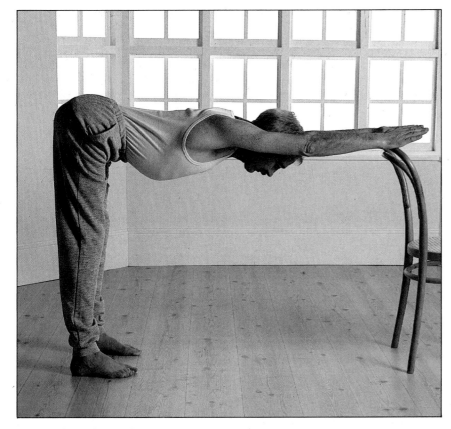

Stretch for a flat back

Tight back-thigh muscles (hamstrings) often contribute to a flat back. To stretch your hamstrings, stand with feet apart and legs straight. Bend forward so your hands touch the back of a chair. Lift your bottom toward the ceiling (photo at left). You should feel a slight dip in the back of your waist. (If your hands are too low, your waist will hump up.) Hold for a few seconds, breathing normally. Breathe in, and come up. To help you lift your bottom and hollow your back, bend your knees slightly (photo below).

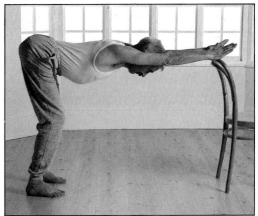

Stretch for a flat back

If you can do the upside-down stretches (see pages 42 to 47), use this position to help your waist to move in correctly. Lie on the floor with your head under the front of a chair. Raise your back and legs so you can rest your knees on the chair seat. Use pillows for comfort, if necessary. Keep your back straight. Hips should be directly above your shoulders. Lift your hips by pressing down on the seat with your knees. Try to pull in the back of your waist at the same time. Hold for a few minutes before bringing your legs down gently.

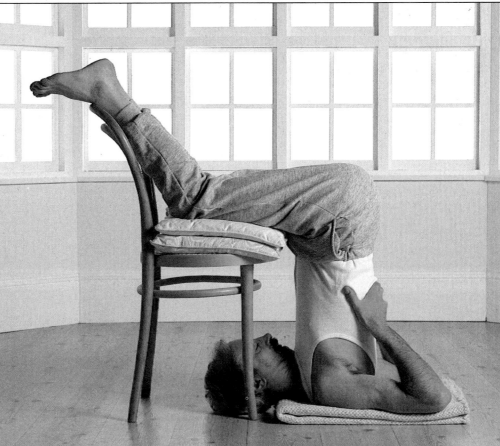

·BACKACHE·

If you have severe backache, don't start stretching without consulting your doctor. Although exercise may form part of your treatment, obtain medical advice first. Specific back problems are discussed on pages 98 and 99.

The cause of most backaches, however, is not easily identifiable. You may have strained a muscle or ligament, there may be pressure on a nerve or you may even be suffering from stress. Daily stretching can prevent and relieve some back pain. In addition to the stretches shown here, all the standing stretches from Chapter One, pages 14 to 47, are good for toning spine and abdominal muscles. The first "less stretch twist" position is also excellent. See page 36.

If your backache is worse at the end of the day, you may need to relax before stretching. If so, lie on your back with your knees bent. See pages 50 and 51. This tilts your pelvis backward and eases pressure on your lower back. Practice deep breathing, (see pages 54 and 55) and let the day's tensions dissolve.

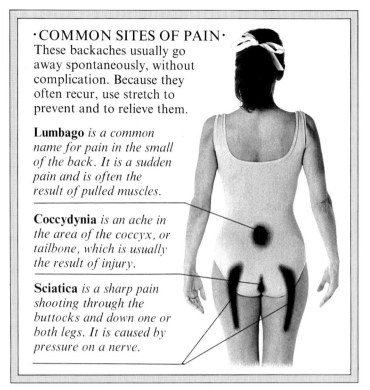

·COMMON SITES OF PAIN·
These backaches usually go away spontaneously, without complication. Because they often recur, use stretch to prevent and to relieve them.

Lumbago *is a common name for pain in the small of the back. It is a sudden pain and is often the result of pulled muscles.*

Coccydynia *is an ache in the area of the coccyx, or tailbone, which is usually the result of injury.*

Sciatica *is a sharp pain shooting through the buttocks and down one or both legs. It is caused by pressure on a nerve.*

First stretch
This stretch eases low backache by toning the muscles of the buttocks, abdomen and thighs.

After relaxing, stay on your back with your knees bent and arms at your sides (photo at top right). Tighten buttock muscles, and raise hips off the floor (photo at bottom right). The lift should come from your hips, not your waist, and your pelvis should be higher than your navel. Keep your chin tucked in straight. Hold for as long as you can, breathing normally. Then breathe out as you slowly uncurl, lowering your hips gently to the floor.

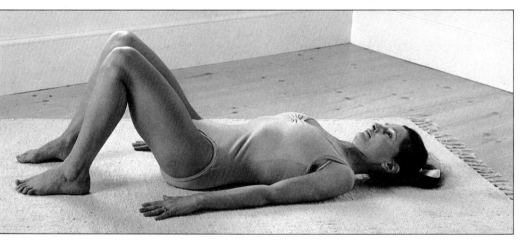

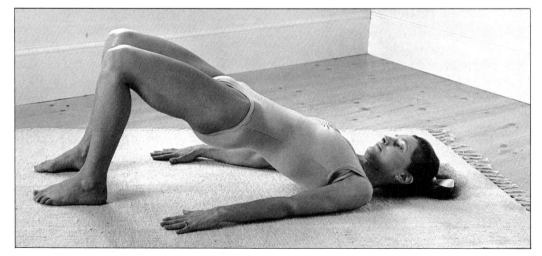

Second stretch

You need a few books for this stretch. Lie on the floor, with knees bent, and keep your back flat and your tailbone tucked in. Tighten the muscles underneath your buttocks. Then stretch your arms above your head to lengthen your upper back. Hold the books to weigh your hands down (photo at top right). Stretch as hard as you can without arching your back. You should feel your abdominal muscles firm and flatten. Still stretching, straighten your legs (photo at bottom right). If you feel any lower-back discomfort, return legs to bent-knee position. If you feel any lower-back discomfort, return legs to bent-knee position. Hold for as long as you can, breathing normally.

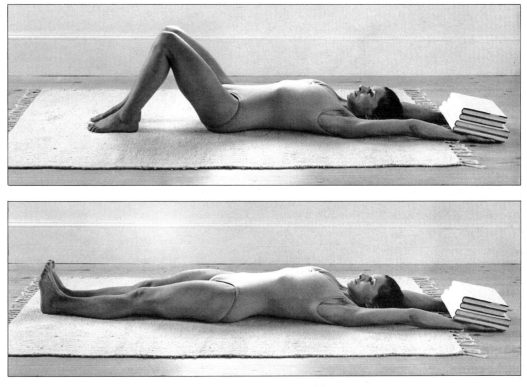

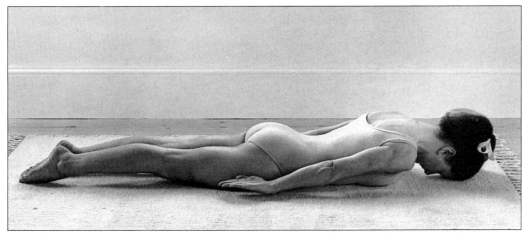

Third stretch

This stretch eases very low backache. Lie on the floor on your face, with arms at your sides, palms up (photo at top left). Follow the instructions on page 40. Don't take your head higher than your feet (photo at bottom left). You should feel the stretch in the sacral region. Hold for a few seconds, breathe out and come down.

To make the stretch more intense, do it with knees bent and shins perpendicular to the floor. Start with your thighs apart, and try to bring your knees together. (This is not shown.)

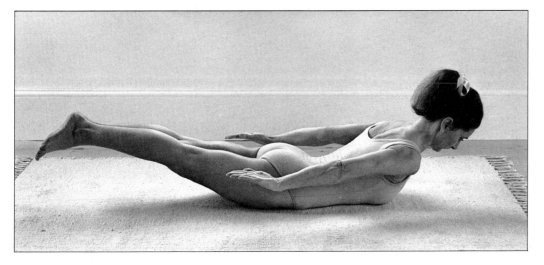

·BACK·PROBLEMS·

Three common back problems are shown here, along with some suggestions for stretches you may find helpful. These stretches should be done by extending and stretching as a whole. This is because a deviation or injury in one particular part of the back affects the entire structure of your body. When you stretch to relieve a specific problem, continue to stretch your entire spine. However, if you have a specific back problem, seek medical advice before you begin.

Scoliosis
Scoliosis is a sideways curvature of the spine. The pelvis tilts to one side. A sideways bend of the spine occurs in the pelvic area, with a compensating curve developing on the opposite side of the upper back. This creates an S-shape. When the problem is severe, it's hard to remedy, and orthopedic treatment may be necessary. If you suffer from severe scoliosis, consult your doctor before you start to stretch.

Many people suffer from scoliosis, to a lesser degree. If your muscles are stronger on one side, depending on whether you are right- or left-handed, you may develop a slight postural imbalance. This can be corrected by stretching both sides of your body evenly. Concentrate on the "less-stretch" movements, so you can extend your spine and stretch the underdeveloped muscles on the weak side of your body. It's ideal if someone can use a pole to check your alignment. See pages 74 to 89.

·PROLAPSED DISK·
Flexible disks are made of cartilage, and they lie between the vertebrae to cushion the bone and allow spinal movement. Disks do not have nerves or blood. But they can cause acute pain if they "prolapse", perhaps because you're overstraining your spine. A *prolapsed disk* (right), more commonly known as a *slipped disk*, requires medical attention. However, standing straight and stretching correctly in most of the positions is still beneficial.
Caution: Avoid all forward stretches if your condition is acute because bending forward can increase pressure on the affected nerve. For the same reason, don't do the basic upside-down stretch; do the "less-stretch upside-down" movement instead.

Scoliotic posture

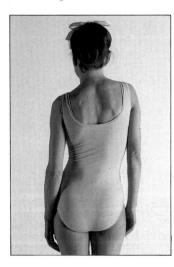

Correcting scoliosis (photo at right)
It is important to stretch correctly in the twists. Ask a friend to hold a pole vertically behind you in one of the "less-stretch" positions to make sure you turn without aggravating the scoliosis. See pages 86 and 87. Listen to your body. If you feel any pain, over and above a normal resistance, make the stretch less intense.

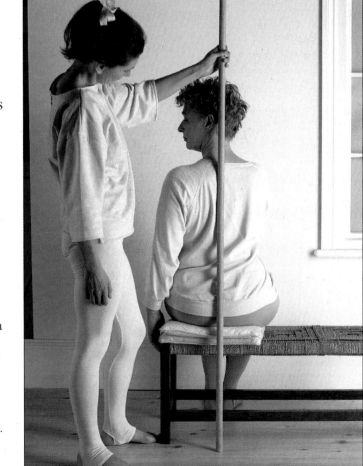

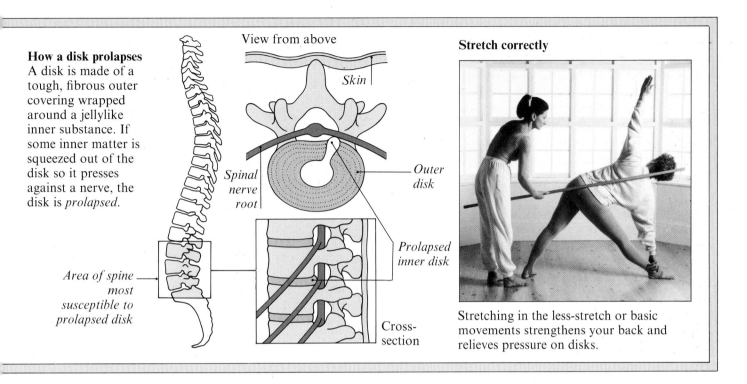

How a disk prolapses
A disk is made of a tough, fibrous outer covering wrapped around a jellylike inner substance. If some inner matter is squeezed out of the disk so it presses against a nerve, the disk is *prolapsed*.

Area of spine most susceptible to prolapsed disk

View from above

Skin

Spinal nerve root

Outer disk

Prolapsed inner disk

Cross-section

Stretch correctly

Stretching in the less-stretch or basic movements strengthens your back and relieves pressure on disks.

Kyphosis

Kyphosis is an outward curve of the upper spine that causes hunched, rounded shoulders. It is often the result of degenerating vertebrae, muscles and ligaments in old age.

If you have kyphosis, the outward curve of your upper back makes your neck curve in and your head drop forward. When you stretch, try to extend the back of your neck so the back of your skull comes into line. All the stretches in Chapter One are beneficial, especially the twists. See pages 34 to 37. When relaxing, put a pillow under your head. See page 52.

Correcting kyphosis
Lie on the floor with a folded blanket or rug under your shoulders and elbows. With knees bent and feet on the seat of a chair, hold the front legs of the chair (photo below left). Take a few deep breaths. On an out-breath, press your feet down on the front of the chair seat, and lift your hips (photo below right). Stretch your spine, extend your neck and tuck in your chin. Keep shoulder blades tucked in to give extra support and to increase the stretch. Use your feet to lift your hips so your upper back extends and straightens. Hold for a few seconds, breathing normally. Breathe out, come down and repeat once or twice.

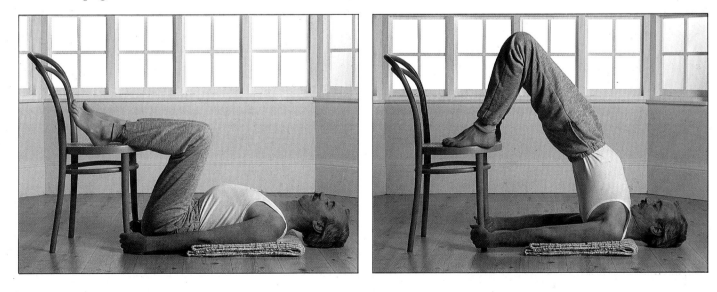

·UPPER·BODY·

The upper body consists of the head, the neck, the shoulders, the upper back, the arms and the hands. The upper body is an extremely mobile structure and is vulnerable to distortion by muscular tension.

If the weight of the head is carried correctly on top of the spine, the neck can move freely. However, often the head is carried slightly off balance. Muscles on one side of the neck tighten. As a result, tightness around the neck and shoulders can cause breathing problems and affect movement of arms and hands.

When you stand properly, with shoulders free and your chest open, your arms and hands relax, and you use your fingers and wrists with ease. When you are stiff across the shoulders and neck, your hands and wrists feel tight and tense. To ease stiffness, look at the stretches on the following 5 pages.

·STRUCTURE OF THE UPPER BODY·

The bony upper body is lighter and more mobile than the weight-supporting hips, legs and lower spine. The vertebrae become smaller at the top of the spine, allowing the neck to turn easily. The shoulder girdle is attached by ligaments at the thorax, only where the collarbones meet the top of the breastbone, allowing it to glide freely over the ribcage. The ribcage is elastic; the curving ribs, which hang from the spine at the back, attach to the breastbone through cartilage. This enables the ribcage to expand and contract with breathing.

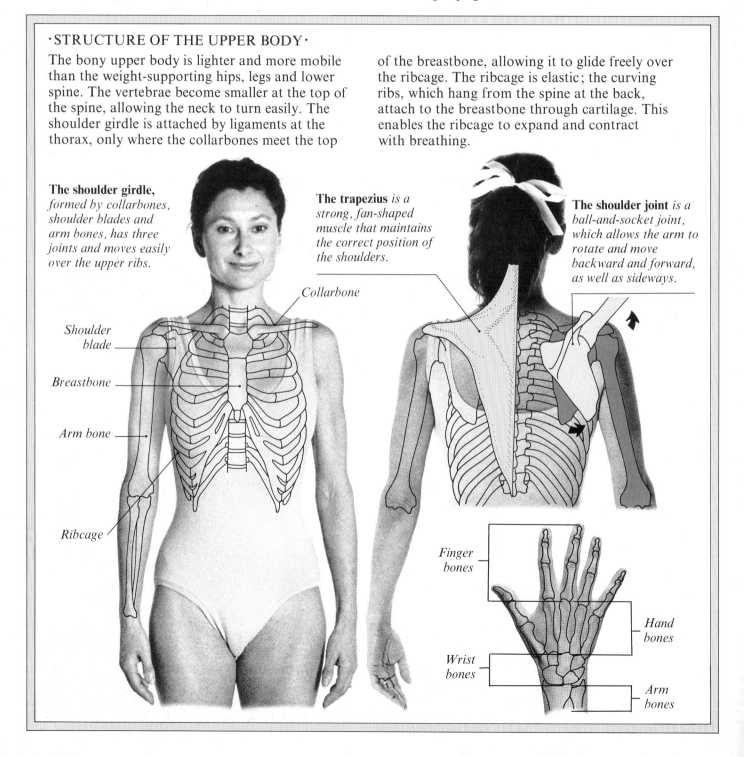

The shoulder girdle, *formed by collarbones, shoulder blades and arm bones, has three joints and moves easily over the upper ribs.*

The trapezius *is a strong, fan-shaped muscle that maintains the correct position of the shoulders.*

The shoulder joint *is a ball-and-socket joint, which allows the arm to rotate and move backward and forward, as well as sideways.*

Collarbone

Shoulder blade

Breastbone

Arm bone

Ribcage

Finger bones

Wrist bones

Hand bones

Arm bones

·HEAD & NECK·

The way you habitually hold your head affects the amount of wear on the small vertebrae and disks in your neck. Often your neck muscles tighten. Tension in the neck is a common cause of headache.

If your neck is stiff, you'll find the sideways stretches and twists difficult. Relieve tension by doing one or more of the movements on this page before you do your usual stretch program. Be sure you use a thick, folded blanket under your shoulders in the upside-down stretches. When relaxing, use a small pillow under your head.

First stretch
Kneel on all fours. Lift your bottom up and extend your spine. Straighten your arms and legs. Let your chest open and your shoulders stretch. Keep your abdominal muscles firm. Let your head hang freely. Keep your throat and face relaxed. Hold for 1 minute before returning to all fours.

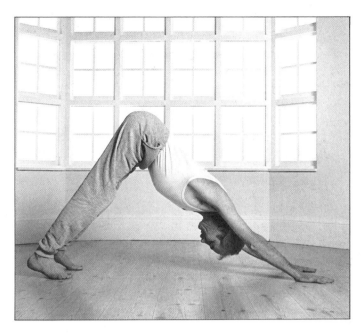

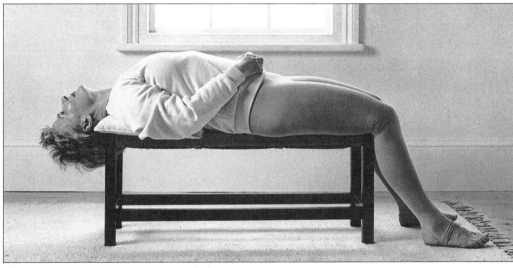

Second stretch
This stretch can be done lying on a bed or low table. Lie so the back of your head is just off the edge of the table. Use a pillow to extend the curve of your neck. You should feel a gentle stretch in your neck but no tension in your eyes or forehead. Hold for 1 minute; support your head with your hands as you come up.

Third stretch
This "more-stretch forward" movement is excellent to let the weight of your head help stretch your neck. See page 33. Either hold your elbows (photo at far right) or let your arms hang down heavily from the shoulders (photo at right). Hold for 1 minute, breathe in and come up.

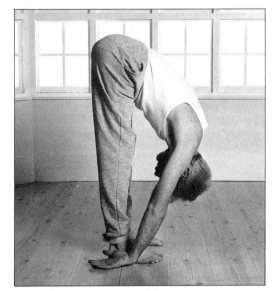

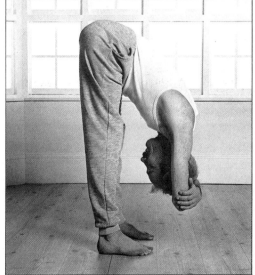

·SHOULDERS·

The shoulder joints are the most mobile joints in your body. They consist of collarbones at the front, arm bones, and shoulder blades at the back, allowing your arms to move in almost any direction. See page 100. Problems frequently arise because over a period of time this range of movement becomes restricted.

A rounded back and stiff shoulders are often the result of poor posture over many years. Most occupations require a lot of forward bending, as people stoop over desks, workbenches, babies, drawing boards or kitchen sinks. The tendency when bending forward with the neck unsupported is to tighten the trapezius muscle (the strong fan-shaped muscle behind the top of the shoulders and neck – see page 100). You may find yourself doing this without noticing it, to stop yourself tilting forward. After a time this tightening of the neck and shoulders becomes a habit, and the muscle fails to release completely even when you are no longer bending forward. After awhile your whole upper body and neck may become distorted.

In many older people there is an increase in the curve of the upper back. This causes the shoulders to push forward and the chest to cave in. Tension in the shoulders then hinders the movement of the ribs and affects breathing. See page 55.

Once established, the habit of tightening your shoulders is extremely difficult to correct. It becomes second nature to round your shoulders every time you stand or sit. The stretches on these pages have been designed to loosen stiffness in the muscles slowly, gradually restoring a full range of movement. Do the whole range of stretches every day immediately before your regular practice session. See pages 58 to 73. Practice the movements slowly and carefully, aiming to increase your range. The shoulders should *never* be forced or wrenched. If you have ever injured or dislocated your shoulders, consult your doctor before doing the stretches.

The stretches on the next two pages can all be done standing, or in a sitting position. At first you may feel your muscles tense and tighten as you stretch. Hold each position for a second or two only and then repeat it. As your shoulders become looser you will find you can gradually build up the time you hold each stretch. Start the sequence by relaxing your shoulders as much as you can (photo below). The stretches will come more easily if you take a little time over this first.

Relaxing your shoulders
Kneel on a folded blanket or rug. Let your head rest comfortably on some pillows in front of you, perhaps raised on a low stool. Fold your arms and hold your elbows, leaning forward so your elbows are a bit higher than your head. As you relax forward you will feel a gentle stretch in your shoulders. Do *not* try to press down in this position; simply relax and on every out-breath feel the tension in your shoulders gradually easing.

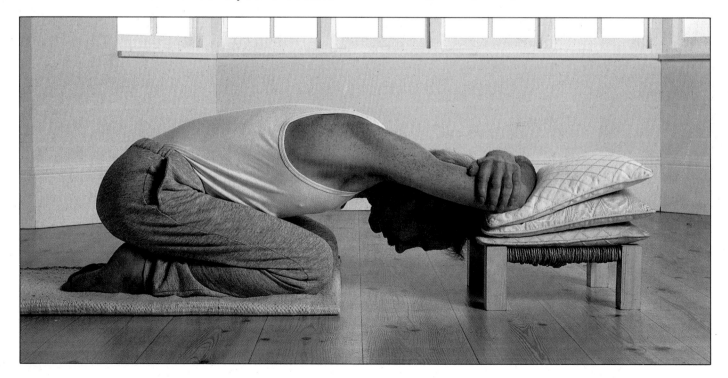

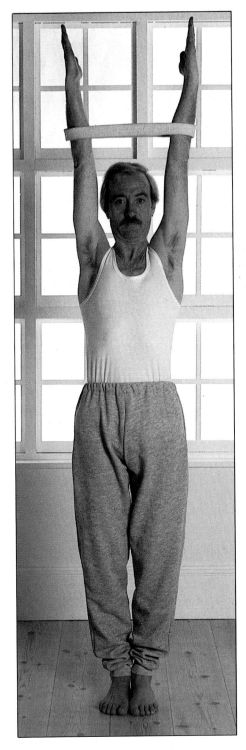

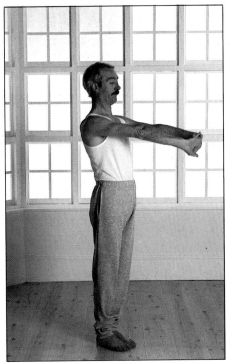

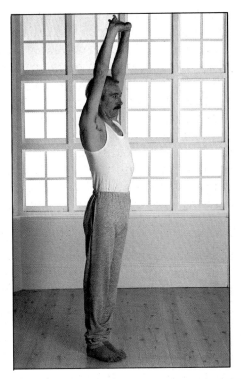

Second stretch

Link your fingers and turn your palms out. Bring your arms up to shoulder level, elbows straight. On a deep out-breath stretch your arms up above your head. Stretch your wrists and open your palms. Repeat with opposite thumb on top.

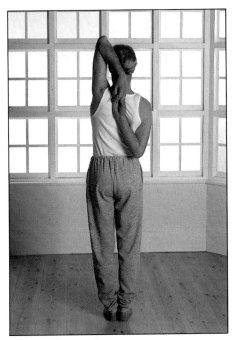

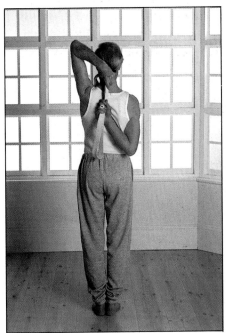

First stretch

Tie a belt around your elbows so when you push against it your elbows are as wide apart as your shoulders. Move your arms above your head, palms facing each other, and keep your elbows straight. Push outward against the belt. You will feel the stretch in your shoulders.

Third stretch

Bend your right elbow so your hand rests vertically on your spine, palm out. Breathing in, stretch your left arm over your head; breathing out, bend your elbow and catch your hands or, if this is hard, a belt. Repeat, hands the other way around.

·SHOULDERS·

Stretching forward
If you are doing a beginners' or basic program,
do these two shoulder stretches sitting as shown. If
you usually do a "more-stretch" program, try
stretching forward standing, keeping your
legs straight.

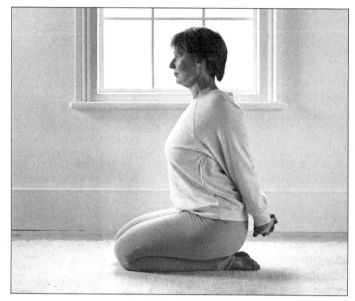

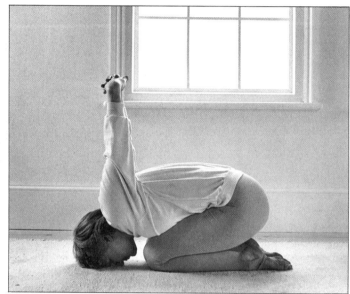

Fourth stretch

1 Kneel and sit on your heels. Clasp your hands together
behind your back. (If this is hard at first, hold a belt
instead.) Open your chest, and straighten your elbows. Take
a few breaths, then breathe in deeply.

2 On an out-breath, bend forward. Keeping your bottom
on your heels, stretch your arms back and up as you go
down. Rest your chest on your thighs. (If your knees are
stiff, put a pillow on your heels under your hips.)

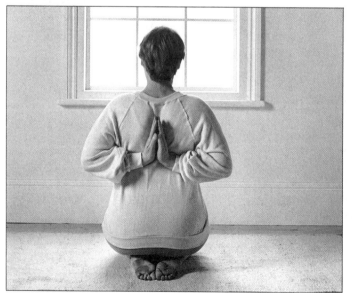

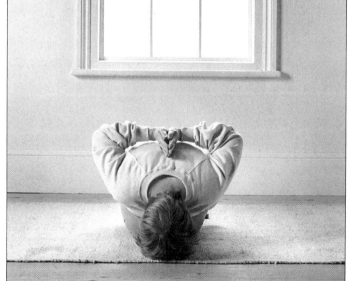

Fifth stretch

1 Place your hands behind your back, with palms together
and fingers pointing down. Then point your fingers up
and try to move your elbows back. Hold for a few seconds.

2 Take a deep breath, and bend forward as you breathe
out. Keep your elbows back so your fingers and thumbs
touch as you go down. Hold for a few seconds, breathing
normally. Breathe in, and come up.

·HANDS·

Your fingers are normally slightly curled when relaxed, and they may stiffen in this position. The stretches on this page will help loosen stiff fingers, hands and wrists. Do them daily for a few months, and your hands will become more flexible.

First stretch

If your fingers are stiff and hard to straighten, they need some help. Gently extend them back, one by one (photo at right). Then stretch them all back at the same time (photo at far right). This helps stretch open your palm. Repeat several times.

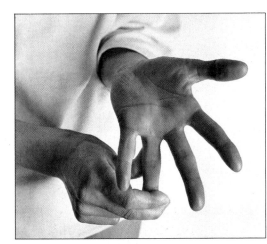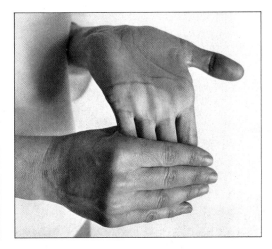

Second stretch

Stretch your thumb back toward your wrist (photo at right). Then bring it forward, stretching gently and firmly (photo at far right). *Never* force it. Finish by making a fist, then slowly opening it. Stretch your fingers and thumb out as far as you can.

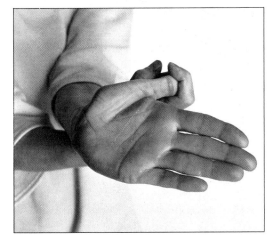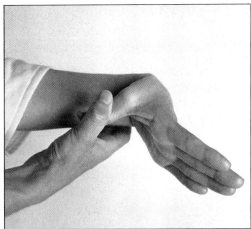

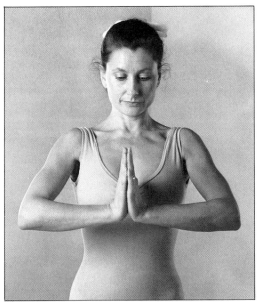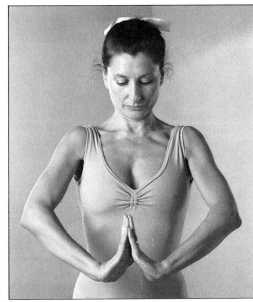

Third stretch

Put your palms together, with fingers pointing upward, as if you were praying. Stretch your fingers, and press palms together strongly. Keep the base of your palms pressing together as you gradually lower your hands until lower arms are horizontal (photo at far left). Then take your hands down farther, with fingers and upper palms together (photo at left). Feel the stretch on the insides of your fingers and wrists. Hold for a few seconds, then repeat.

·HIPS·

If you have flexible hip joints, you shouldn't have difficulty in moving your legs backward and forward, swinging them away from and across your body or rotating them in and out. Without feeling strain on your spine, your pelvis can adjust and support the weight of your upper body as you walk, stand and run.

Unfortunately, freedom of movement in hip joints is a casualty of western civilization. In eastern cultures, people living without furniture, fitted kitchens or bathrooms spend a lot of time squatting and sitting on the floor. Their flexibility and ease of movement are in striking contrast with the stiffness of western adults. Your child may squat happily to play, but if you spend your days sitting in chairs or cars, you quickly lose the ability to rotate your thighs.

During the first half of your life, this may not seem to matter. But hips that are not used fully develop tight muscles. In time, uneven pressure on

joints causes wear and tear, commonly known as *arthritis* or *osteoarthritis*. This leads to farther restricted movement. Stiffness and pain in joints mean you use them even less, and slowly the muscles begin to waste away. It is a vicious circle: use your hip joints properly when you can, or there may come a time when you can't.

Many sports – including jogging, skiing and cycling – involve restricted hip movement. Stretch, on the other hand, actively promotes flexible hips. All the basic stretches from Chapter One help ease stiffness in the muscles surrounding hip joints. (Pay attention to the position of your feet on the floor in the standing stretches. When legs are straight, keep your knees strongly extended to be sure you feel the stretch correctly.) All the stretches on these 3 pages are designed to improve the rotation of the thighs. Stretch will help you maintain flexible hips or loosen stiff ones.

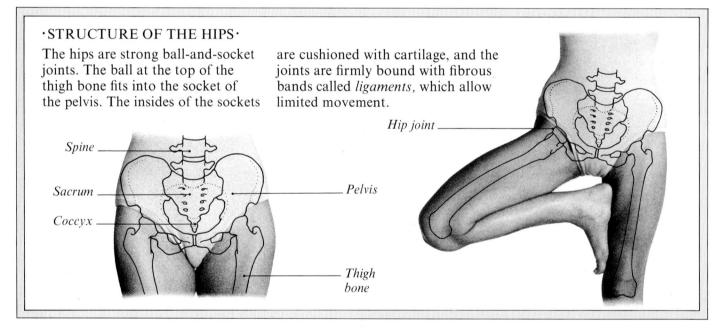

·STRUCTURE OF THE HIPS·

The hips are strong ball-and-socket joints. The ball at the top of the thigh bone fits into the socket of the pelvis. The insides of the sockets are cushioned with cartilage, and the joints are firmly bound with fibrous bands called *ligaments,* which allow limited movement.

Spine

Sacrum

Coccyx

Pelvis

Thigh bone

Hip joint

First stretch
To test the flexibility of your hips and give them a good stretch, lie on your back and bend your knees. Move your feet toward your buttocks, with soles together. Let your knees fall apart. Your weight should be evenly distributed so both knees are the same distance from the floor.

If your knees don't easily fall outward, try this stretch with your feet raised on pillows (photo at right). Have the soles of your feet against each other, and relax into the stretch for a few minutes every day.

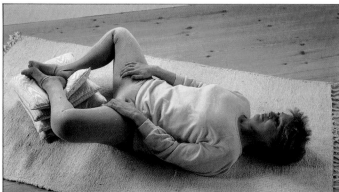

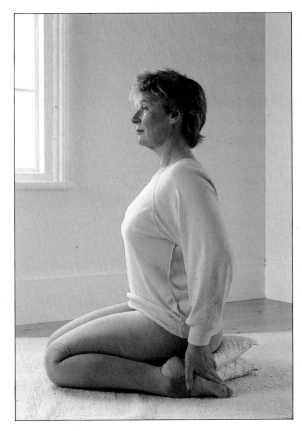

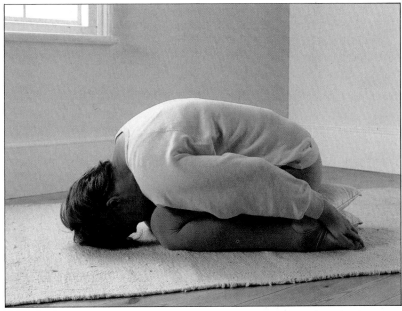

Second stretch
Sit on pillows between your feet. Keep your knees together (photo at left). If this feels easy, try bending forward while keeping your bottom on the floor (photo above). As the position becomes more comfortable, remove one pillow at a time, until after a few weeks you're sitting on the floor.

Third stretch
Sit on the floor, and cross one knee over the other. With your hands on the floor for support, sit as tall as you can. Hold for a few seconds, then repeat with your knees the other way around.

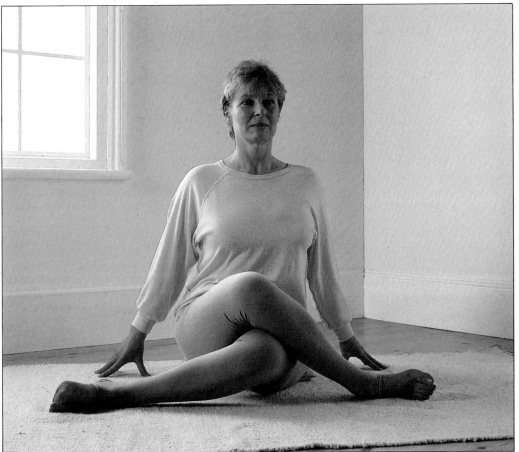

·HIPS·

Stretching upside down

In the upside-down positions, the hip joints don't have to support the weight of your body while you stretch and work them. This is especially useful if you suffer from arthritis in your hips.

Fourth stretch

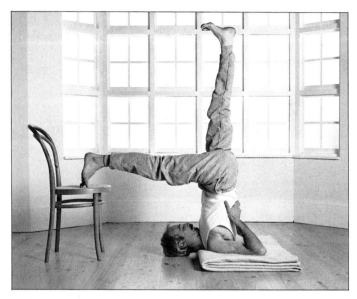

Make your body vertical. Rest your neck and shoulders on a folded rug or blanket. Extend your body in the basic inverted position. As you stretch, lower one leg, and rest your foot on a chair behind your head. Your back and hips should remain straight. Breathe normally. Hold up to 30 seconds, keeping both knees straight. Then stretch both legs up again, and repeat stretch with the other leg. When this becomes easy, move your foot down a little more, onto a stool or pile of books.

Before you try the stretches on this page, you must be able to maintain the basic upside-down position comfortably and securely for 5 minutes. See pages 42 and 43. If possible, ask someone to help position your chair and books.

Fifth stretch

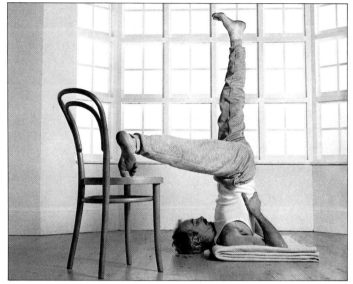

When you have mastered the previous stretch, move your leg out to the side. Start with a straight back and both legs stretching up. Turn one leg out as far as possible before you move it out to the side. Lower it to a chair. How far sideways you move your leg depends on the outward rotation of your thighs. Keep knees straight and your body vertical. Extend lower back, and keep abdominal muscles firm. Breathe normally. Hold up to 30 seconds, then stretch up and repeat with the other leg.

Sixth stretch
Again start with a straight back and both legs stretching up. Keep knees straight. Slowly move both legs out to the side, and lower them onto a low table or two piles of books. Lift your hips, and stretch the backs of your legs. Breathe normally. Hold up to 30 seconds and bend your knees to come up.

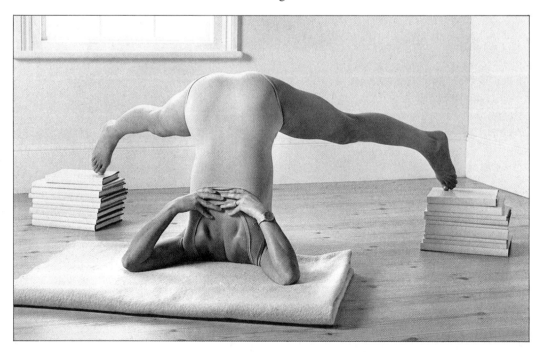

·KNEES & LEGS·

Knees are the most vulnerable parts of your legs, and accidents and injuries are the cause of most knee problems. The construction of the knee is complicated. Crisscrossing ligaments hold the joint in place, while pads of cartilage act as shock absorbers between the bones. If wear and tear on the knee joint is uneven and muscles weaken, a sudden blow or awkward movement can cause the cartilage to slip out of place or even tear. It's also possible to stand so the backs of your legs become overstretched (photo at right).

Stretching is the perfect exercise for knees and legs, but consult your doctor if you ever injured your knees. If your leg muscles are aching and tired by the end of the day, or if you have varicose veins, the upside-down stretches are a wonderful antidote. See pages 42 to 47. The stretches on the next 2 pages are designed to strengthen the muscles around the knees, especially the front-thigh muscles.

·OVERSTRETCHED LEG·

When you stand with legs straight, your weight should fall on the center of your hip joints, knees and ankles (below). If you overstretch your legs as you stand, the extra strain on the backs of your knees weakens ligaments behind them (right).

To correct overstretched legs, keep your weight over the balls of your feet instead of on your heels, and keep knees straight, but not hyperextended. Lift your front thigh muscles, when stretching.

·STRUCTURE OF THE LEG·

The leg consists of four bones. The femur, or thigh bone, connects the hip to the knee. It is the longest, strongest bone in the body. At its lower end, it forms part of the knee joint. A small, flat, triangular bone, the patella (kneecap) makes a hinge at the front that protects the knee joint. Below the knee are two leg bones. The tibia (shin bone) runs from the front of the knee to the ankle and forms part of the knee and ankle joints. The fibula lies on the outer side of the tibia and forms part of the ankle joint at its lower end.

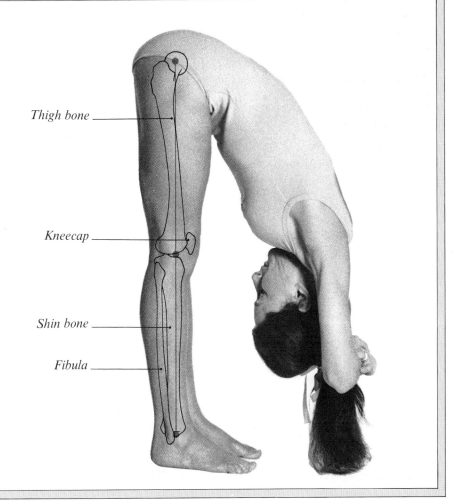

Thigh bone

Kneecap

Shin bone

Fibula

·KNEES & LEGS·

Even if the knee joint has been weakened, it can still be partially protected by strengthening the muscles around it. The three exercises on these pages improve the muscle tone of the thighs.

First stretch

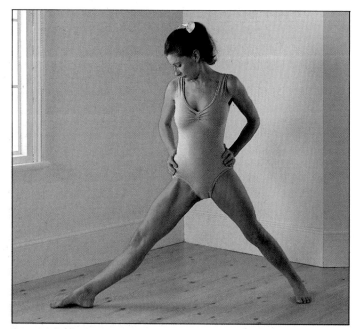

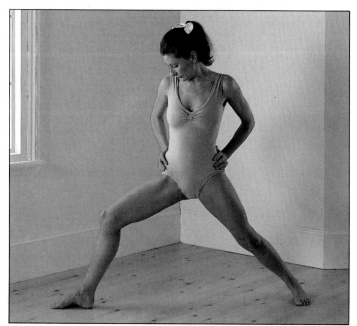

1 With your hands on your hips, spread your feet wide apart. Turn your left foot slightly in and your right leg out. The center of your right knee should face the right, in line with your right foot. Spread out your toes, lift the arch of your right foot. Pull up your right kneecap by tightening your front thigh muscles.

2 Resist with your shin, and bend your right knee a bit. Keep your knee in line with your foot. Hold for a few seconds, pulling up your kneecap. Relax your muscles, and bend your knee a little more. Keep resisting with your shin. Hold for a few more seconds, pulling up your front thigh muscles.

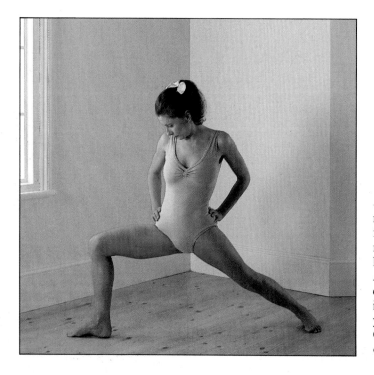

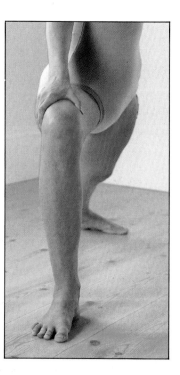

3 Continue to bend your right knee, until your right thigh is parallel to the floor and your shin is at a right angle to it (photo at left). Keep heel flat on floor. At each stage, be sure the center of your knee is still in line with the center of your foot (photo at right). Come up slowly, and repeat on the other side.

Second stretch

Stand with your back against a wall and your
feet slightly in front of you about 6 inches
apart. Your legs should be straight and your
feet parallel to each other pointing forward.
Bend your knees slightly without turning
them out. Keeping your back straight, slide
down the wall a little. Hold for a count of 5.
With your feet still pointing forward, bend
your knees a little more. Again hold for a
count of 5. Keeping your heels down on the
floor and your arches lifted, go down in
stages as far as you can. Then come up slowly
in the same way, holding for a count of 5 at
each pause.

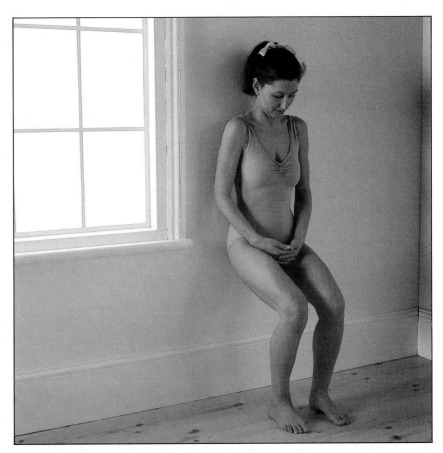

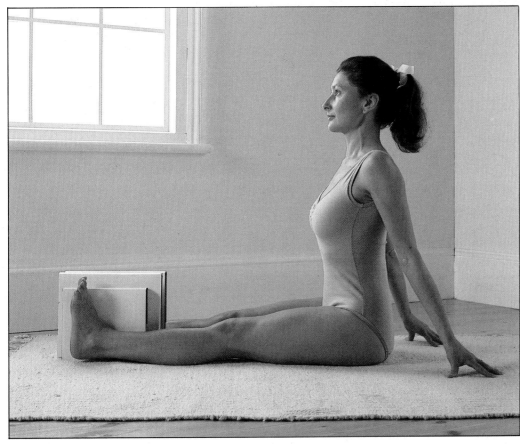

Third stretch

Sit on a rug on the floor,
with back and legs straight
and your hands behind your
back touching the floor for
extra support. (Sit on a
pillow if your lower back
sags.) Stretch your legs, and
extend your heels. If ankles
touch while your knees are
far apart, put a book
between your ankles. Stretch
the insides of your heels and
your big toes to help them
straighten. Tighten front
thigh muscles, and pull up
your kneecaps. Both knees
should be working strongly.
If one side is weaker than
the other, work it a little
harder. Hold for a few
seconds, then relax. Repeat
several times.

·FEET & ANKLES·

Feet should be strong and flexible, with toes evenly spaced so that as you walk they spread out on the floor for balance. Although your feet are a very small base of support for your body, they are well-designed to do the job of bearing your weight. However, it's important to stand correctly, because faults allowed to develop in the feet have postural repercussions throughout your body.

Stand on a dry, smooth surface with wet feet, and see what impression you make. Your toes, heels and soles should press the floor and leave a print. If the print of one foot is better than the other, your weight is not evenly distributed. You should give a little time to standing straight. See page 17. If your arches leave a print, you're suffering from fallen arches. Although flat feet are common in early childhood, in later life fallen arches are frequently the cause of tired, aching feet. This is because your arches hold the bones of your feet and ankles in their correct positions and encourage your foot muscles to function normally. They also act as shock absorbers. If they have fallen, your muscles and ligaments endure extra stress.

Problems with feet are often caused by shoes. Fashion in shoes takes little account of the needs of feet. Even low heels throw body weight forward onto the balls of the feet, making the backs of ankles tight and stiff. Ill-fitting shoes push toes together and may cause corns and calluses to develop. In extreme cases, shoes make toes cross over, and this can inflame the big toe, causing a painful bunion. Women are more prone to almost all foot problems. High heels can throw the body out of line and put excessive pressure on the balls of the feet and the toes, and put the spine under stress.

By stretching your feet, you can help correct the damage done by poor footwear. The stretches shown opposite strengthen the feet.

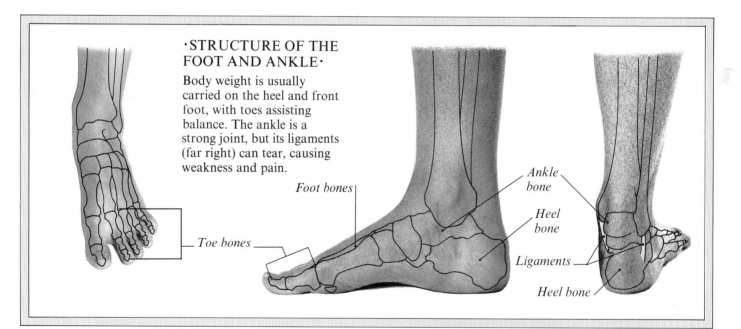

·STRUCTURE OF THE FOOT AND ANKLE·
Body weight is usually carried on the heel and front foot, with toes assisting balance. The ankle is a strong joint, but its ligaments (far right) can tear, causing weakness and pain.

Foot bones

Toe bones

Ankle bone

Heel bone

Ligaments

Heel bone

Caring for your feet
If ill-fitting shoes are deforming your toes, don't wear them. Pull your toes apart with your fingers to stretch them. Put pads of cotton between your toes to keep them separate if necessary (photo at right). Walk with bare feet whenever you can, and always stretch barefoot.

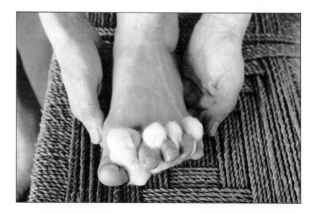

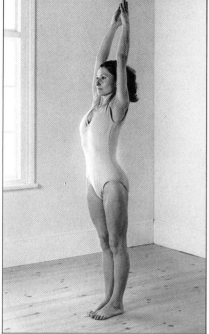

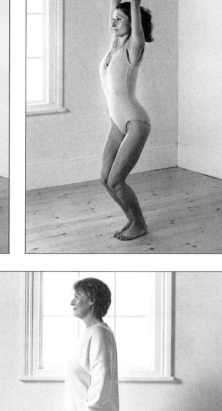

First stretch

This strengthens the muscles of the legs and ankles. Stand up straight, keeping feet parallel and slightly apart. Stretch your arms above your head, with palms together (photo at far left). Take a few breaths. On an out-breath, bend your knees as much as possible, without lifting your heels off the floor or bending forward (photo at left). Extend your lower back and keep your abdominal muscles firm. Breathe in, and come up. Repeat two or three times.

Second stretch

Kneel with feet and ankles together (photo at right). Sit on your heels (photo at far right). If this is difficult, tie a belt around your ankles to keep them from separating. Stretch up through your spine, keeping your weight evenly distributed between your heels. Hold for a few minutes. If fallen arches make your feet ache, do this exercise every day.

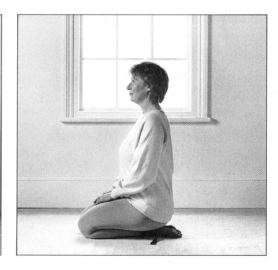

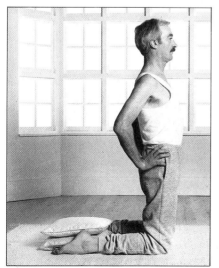

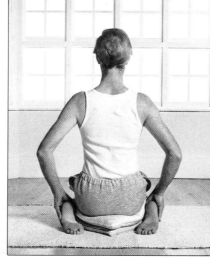

Third stretch

This benefits your arches and strengthens your ankles. Kneel with knees together and pillows between your feet (photo at far left). Sit on the pillows and stretch up through your spine. Then stretch the outsides of your feet toward the floor (photo at left). Hook your thumbs inside your ankles, and turn out your calves. Encourage your little toes to stretch toward the floor. Hold for a few seconds, and repeat as necessary.

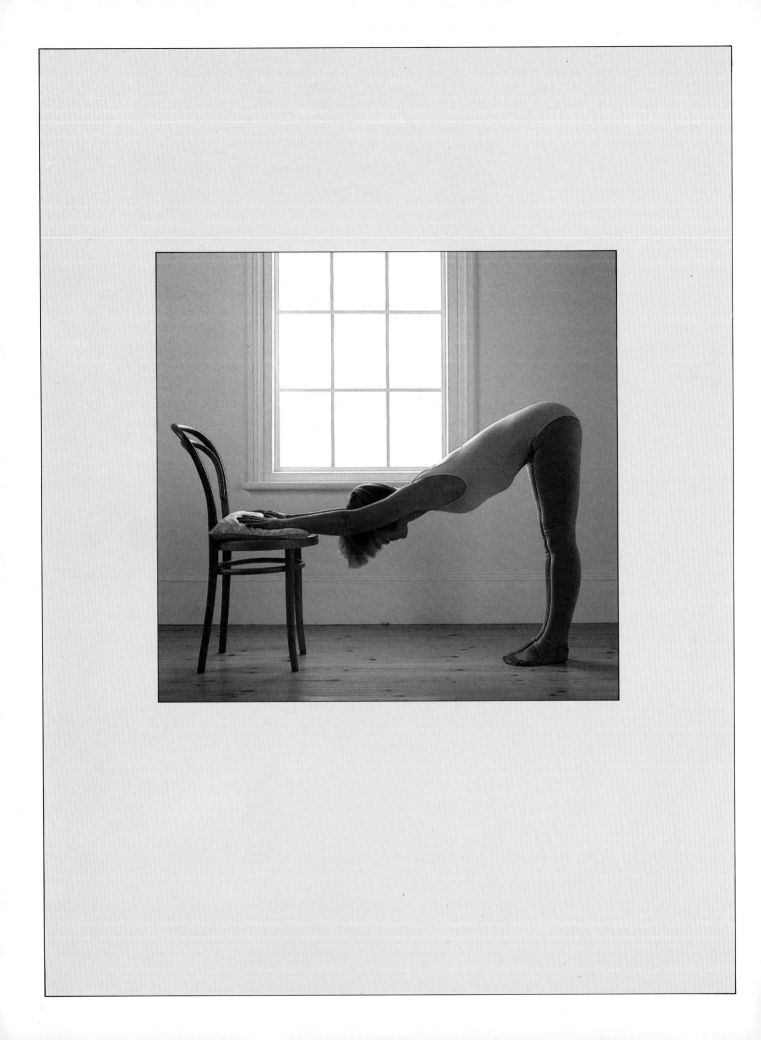

·RELIEVING·STRESS·

Because stress and stress-related problems receive a good deal of publicity, it is easy to forget that a certain amount of stress is necessary. Stress triggers the energy to create, achieve and survive. These responses originated with primitive man who, when alerted to danger, tensed his muscles and quickened his heart rate, preparing for "flight or fight".

Today, it's rarely immediate physical danger that causes fear or anxiety. More often the bus is late, there is pressure at work or personal relationships are difficult. In these circumstances, you may feel the effects of stress but not the release through physical action that your body expects to follow the tension. As anxiety and frustration build, each crisis makes an overstressed person more vulnerable.

Life doesn't run smoothly all the time. Occasionally everyone needs help with physical, mental or emotional stress, and there are many forms of stress relief. Clever marketing convinces people of the need for external remedies – whether in the form of pills, alcohol or therapy. In fact, many crises can be surmounted without resorting to external remedies. Helping yourself from your own resources makes you stronger and better able to cope the next time.

With some time and patience, you can alleviate stress in all its different forms. You may be powerless to solve the problems, but you can do a great deal to keep them from overwhelming you. It may take little to brighten your outlook. For a start, reverse the syndrome of physical tensions caused by emotional setbacks or hostile circumstances. The programs in this chapter are designed to help you respond constructively to various types of crisis and tension.

You should be familiar with the stretches in the first chapter before you do any of these programs because detailed instructions for stretches described in Chapter One are not repeated here. Pay attention to the information in the programs because relieving stress by exercise is more subtle than ordinary everyday stretching.

NOTE: If a picture in this chapter shows a more-advanced stretch from Chapter One than the one you would normally do, replace it by the appropriate movement at your usual stretch level. The benefits will be the same.

·STOP·CRYING·

Everybody cries sometimes. Occasional tears are not bad, but there always comes a time when you have to dry your eyes and get on with life. Often this isn't easy because you find yourself sobbing and gulping long after you want to stop.

By doing some strong, outward stretches, you can keep yourself from being overwhelmed by your emotions as you calm down. The following positions will help you feel more able to face the world again.

1 Relax

Lie on your back, with your body raised off the floor (such as on a low table), while your head and the tops of your shoulders are supported on the floor by pillows. Keep chin tucked in. Breathe slowly and deeply. Keep your eyes open, and fix your gaze on a point above you. Stay in this position for 5 to 10 minutes. To come out of the position, bend your knees and rest a few seconds. Slide your back gently off the stool.

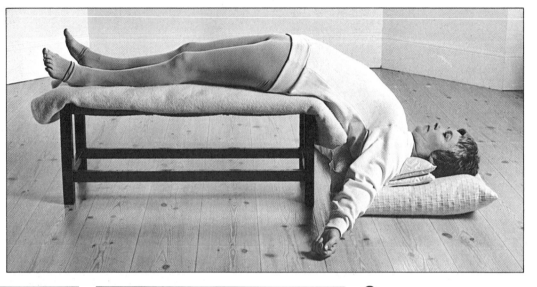

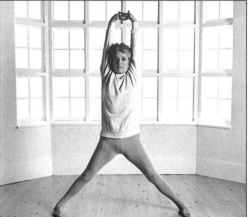

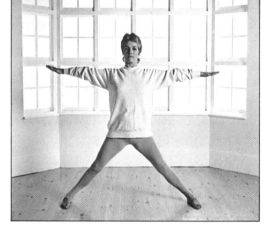

2 Wide and strong

When you feel calm enough to do some active stretching, stand up and do as many stretches as you can shown on pages 22 to 25. (Omit only the second stretch on page 25 because balancing on one leg is not helpful). Hold each position for a few seconds, and change sides when appropriate. Stretch outward strongly. Concentrate on breathing smoothly and steadily. Open your chest as you breathe in deeply. Repeat several times. Your shoulders should feel relaxed before you attempt the next positions.

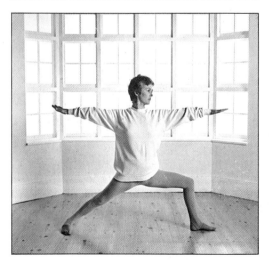

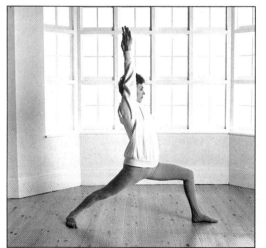

3 Upside down

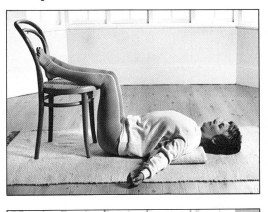

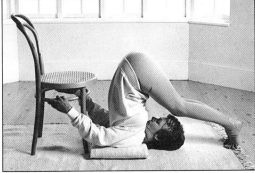

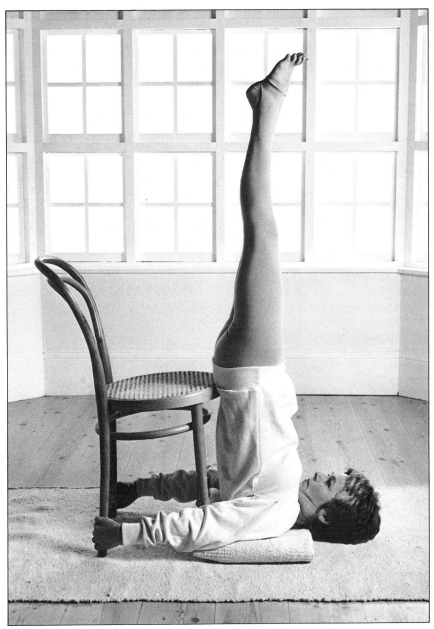

Lie on a rug on the floor, with a folded blanket under your shoulders and upper arms. Keep chin tucked under. Rest your legs on a chair (photo at top). Hold the chair, and pull it toward you as, on an out-breath, you swing your legs over your head. Lift your upper back as much as possible (photo above). Place your feet as far back on the chair as you comfortably can. Pull the chair closer until you can hold its back legs. The seat should support your lower back when you bring your legs above your head, as on pages 42 to 43 (photo at right). Hold up to 5 minutes; come down slowly.

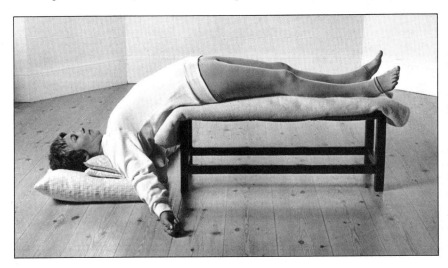

4 Relax

After finishing these active stretches, it's essential to keep your outlook positive. For this reason, don't end by relaxing with your eyes closed. If you want to rest, repeat the first position, with your body raised off the floor. Keep your chest and your eyes open. Breathe slowly and deeply, making your in-breath long and steady. Stay in the position for 5 to 10 minutes before bending your knees. Rest for a few seconds with your feet close to your hips, then slide your back gently down off the stool.

·BANISHING·DEPRESSION·

When you're depressed, you probably stand with your chest caved in, your shoulders drooping and your head down. This posture makes it difficult to look up and face the world, especially as tension builds in upper shoulders. Simple stretches that counteract this postural tendency can make you feel better, whether you've felt miserable for a short time or a long time. However, if your depression is long-standing, carry out this program at least once every day.

1 Shoulders

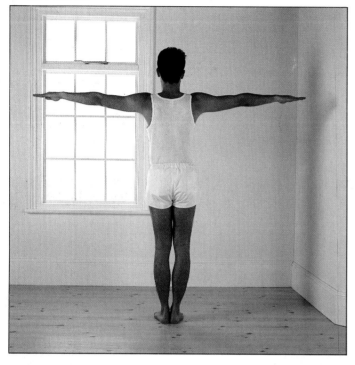

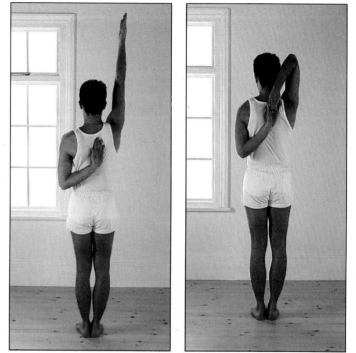

Stand straight and stretch tall. Spread your arms out to the side and stretch away from your body (photo above). Then do the third stretch on page 103 (photo above right). Look up and breathe deeply as you stretch. The straighter you stand, the easier it will be to catch your hands. Repeat this stretch on each side at least twice.

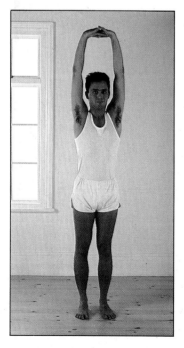

2 Straight

Link your fingers together and turn your palms out. Take your arms up over your head and stretch as tall as you can. Extend the lower back and keep the abdominal muscles firm. Hold for a few seconds and repeat, with fingers linked the other way.

3 Sideways

Extend your spine by doing one of the stretches described on pages 18 to 21. Be careful not to bend forward. As you stretch to the side, open your chest so you can breathe in deeply.

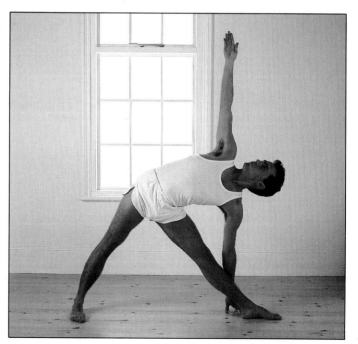

4 Wide and strong

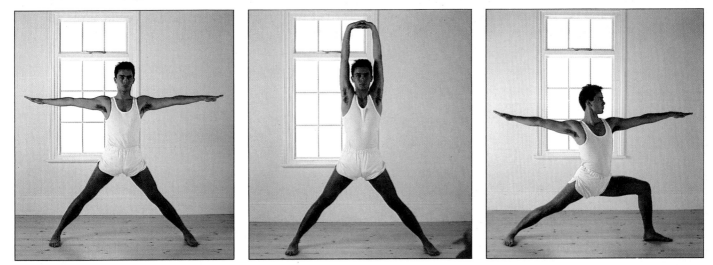

Now do three of the stretches described on pages 22 to 25. Choose them according to your usual level of practice. As you stretch, keep both feet firmly planted on the ground.

Spread your toes, and lift the arches of your feet. This gives you a feeling of stability. Repeat the stretches at least once, and alternate sides when appropriate.

5 Backward

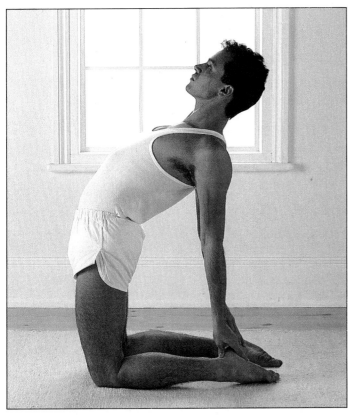

After you have opened your chest and released your shoulders, kneel on a rug, and do one of the stretches described on pages 38 to 41. Hold the position for a few seconds, then sit on your heels to rest.

6 Relax

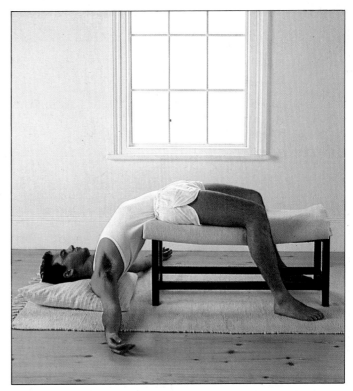

Lie on your back, with your trunk raised on a low table. Head and shoulders are supported by a pillow on the floor. Bend your knees, and place feet flat on the floor or raised on a low stool. Keep your eyes open; hold this position for at least 5 minutes. Then slide your back down to the floor, and rest for a few seconds before you stand up.

·RENEWING·ENERGY·

You may not express openly anger and anxiety with your body. Instead, you're more likely to repress irritation and react to the frustrations that build during the day by tightening muscles. If you end a working day full of frustration and aggression, you can't get going again until you get rid of your negative feelings. This stretch program will ease the day's tensions and leave you feeling relaxed and energetic.

1 Lie down

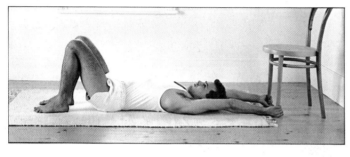

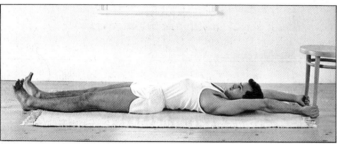

Lie on your back on a rug in front of a chair. Bend your knees, and keep your feet flat on the floor. Keep chin tucked in. Reach your arms over your head, and grasp the chair legs firmly (top photo). Extend into your heels as you push the chair away from you (photo above). Breathe deeply, then release the chair, and rest for a second or two. Repeat.

2 Legs raised

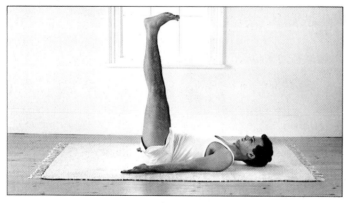

Bring your arms down by your sides, and bend your knees, sinking your pelvis into the floor. Without arching your back, raise your legs over your waist, then straighten them. Hold for a few seconds before bending your knees and bringing legs down, breathing out as you do so.

3 On your side

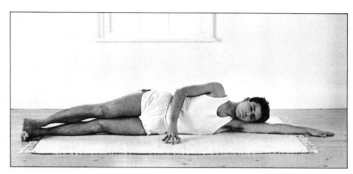

Next bring your legs down, and turn onto your left side. Stretch out your left arm, and extend the whole of the left side of your body from heel to fingertips.

4 On your side

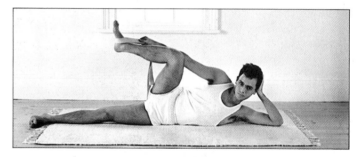

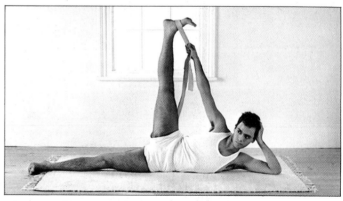

Support your head with your left hand. Loop a belt around your right foot, and hold it. Keep your right knee bent (top photo). Then straighten your knee, and raise your right leg (photo above). Hold for a few seconds before bringing your leg down. If it's hard to keep your body in line, practice against a wall. Roll over, and repeat steps 3 and 4 on the other side.

5 On all fours

Turn on your front, and kneel on all fours, with your hands and feet body-width apart (photo at right). Breathing out, straighten your legs, and raise your bottom as high as you can on your tiptoes (photo at far right). Keep your spine and legs stretched. Take your heels down toward the floor (photo at below right). Keep your chest open and your neck relaxed to get rid of stiffness in upper shoulders. Hold for a few seconds before returning to all fours.

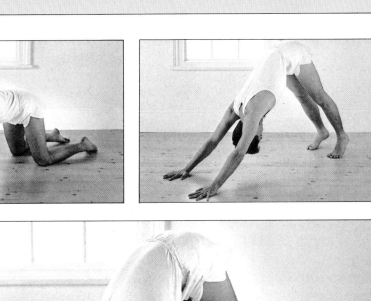

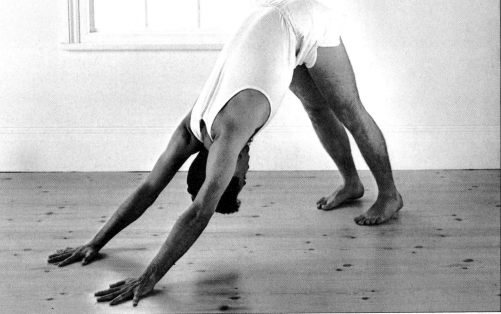

6 Reach out

Stand straight, and stretch up through your spine. Do one sideways stretch (photo below) and one wide-and-strong stretch (photo below right) described on pages 18 to 25.

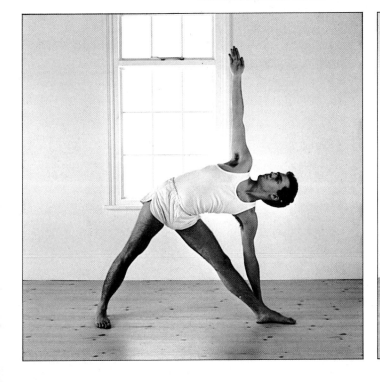

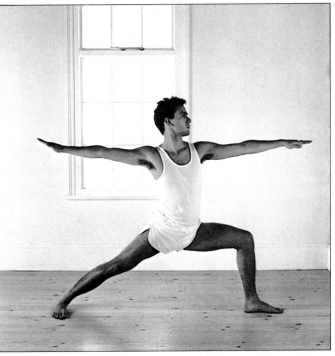

·RECOVERING·FROM·A·JOURNEY·

Traveling often involves sitting in cramped conditions for long periods of time, whether in a car, train or plane. After being confined in a small space for hours, you are unlikely to relax easily when the journey is over. Additional tensions caused by driving in heavy traffic or waiting at airports make unwinding even more difficult. This program will relieve travel-related stress and can be done as soon as your journey is over.

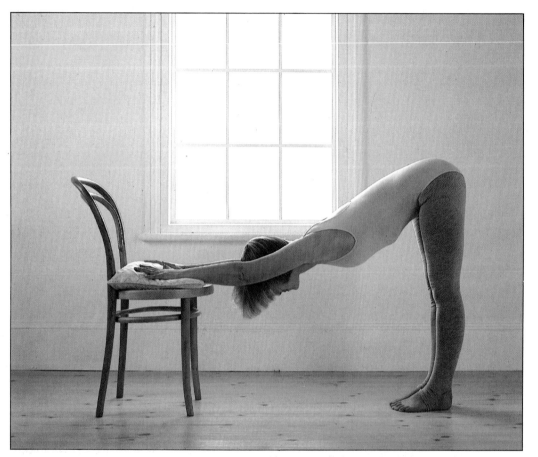

1 Forward

Stand near a chair, and do the first forward stretch described on page 32. Bend from your hips, keeping legs straight but not hyper-extended. Concentrate on reaching forward and stretching your shoulders and the backs of your legs. Take your hands down only as far as you can manage without curving your back. Each time you breathe out, try to take your chest a little closer to the floor. Hold for up to 1 minute.

2 Twist

Kneel down on a rug with your knees together, and sit on your heels. Interlock your fingers, and breathe out as you stretch your arms above your head. Turn palms up (photo at right). Take a few breaths before bringing your arms down. On the next out-breath, twist around as far as step 3 of the basic stretch, shown on page 34. Keep your shoulders relaxed (photo at far right). Hold for a few seconds before stretching up and twisting around to the other side. Maintain the lift in your spine.

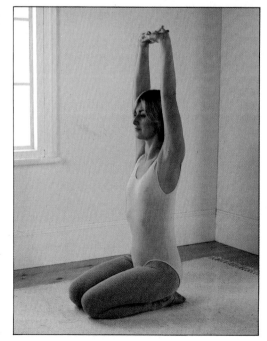

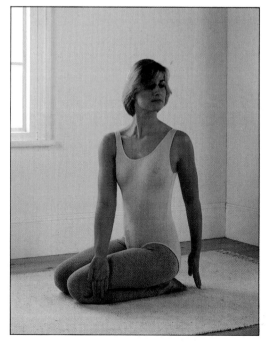

3 Straight

With knees together, take your feet apart, and sit between your heels (photo at right). (If you are stiff and this is difficult, put a pillow under your buttocks.) Put your hands behind your back, and link your fingers (photo at far right). Sitting straight, relax your shoulders. Let your hands drop toward the floor while you open your chest and breathe deeply. Hold for up to 5 minutes.

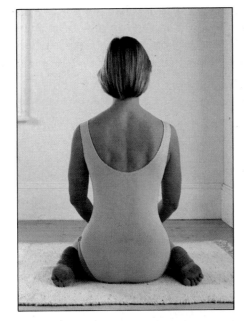 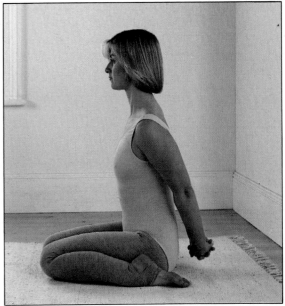

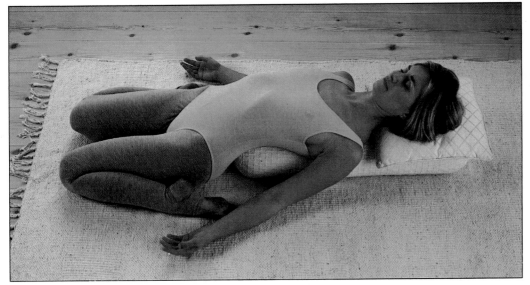

4 Backward

If you're comfortable sitting between your heels, lie back on the floor and stretch the front of your thighs. If your front thigh muscles are very tight – from walking, cycling or skiing – you will be more comfortable lying on a large pillow. Ten minutes lying in this position is extremely relaxing.
Caution: If you have a history of knee or lower back problems, do the relaxation position at the top of page 53 with your body raised up on pillows.

5 Relax

Lie on a rug on the floor, and relax as described on pages 50 and 51. Concentrate on making your out-breath long and slow, easing tension in your shoulders and hips. Stay in this position for 10 to 15 minutes.

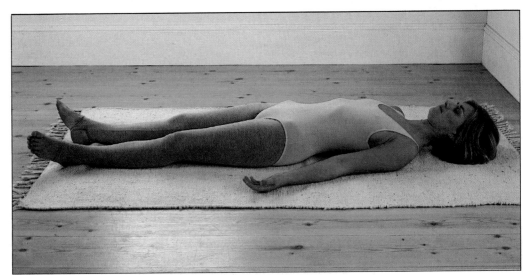

·CALMING·DOWN·

Some days the telephone never stops, and home or the office demand reserves you don't have. By the end of such a day, you may feel exhausted yet unable to calm down. Your mind is so active you can't relax; your body is tired and tight with fatigue so deep breathing is useless. This program will help your muscles to relax and your mind to slow down. Gradually you will begin to breathe quietly and deeply.

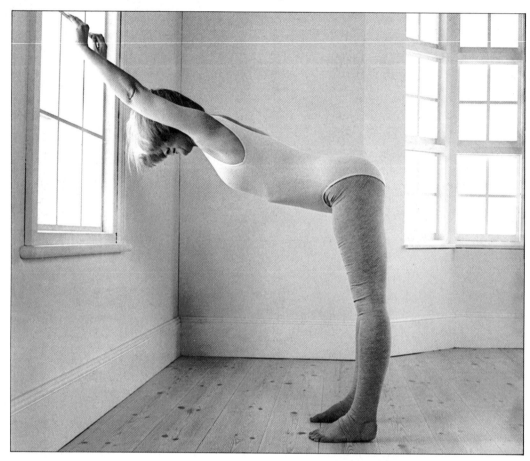

1 Up and forward

Stand with feet 6 inches apart. Stretch up and forward until your hands are resting on a high shelf or window sash. Breathe out, and feel your spine stretch from your tailbone toward your head. Continue to breathe slowly; after each out-breath feel the tension ease in your shoulders and upper back. Hold for up to 1 minute.

2 Straight

Stand straight. Link your fingers together, palms out. As you breathe in, extend arms to shoulder level. As you breathe out, move them above your head. Breathe deeply, and maintain the stretch in your spine (photo at right). Keep your feet firmly planted on the floor, with toes spread out, and feel yourself stretch very tall. Hold for a few seconds. Breathing out, let your arms drop and relax your shoulders (photo at far right). Stand straight, and breathe deeply and slowly for 1 or 2 minutes without straining.

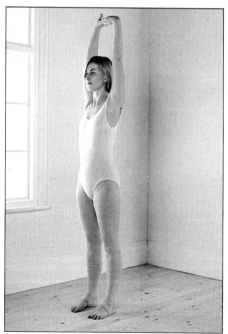

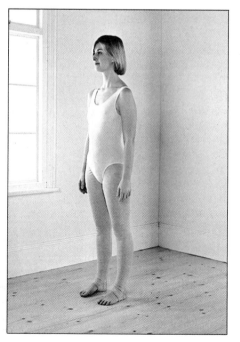

3 On all fours

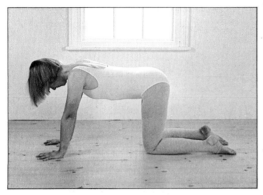

Kneel on all fours (photo above). On an out-breath, straighten your legs and move your hips back and up. Keep your back straight. Then take your heels down to the floor (photo at right). Hold for up to 30 seconds, then come back on all fours.

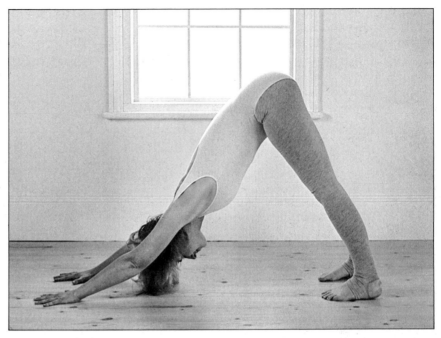

4 Shoulders

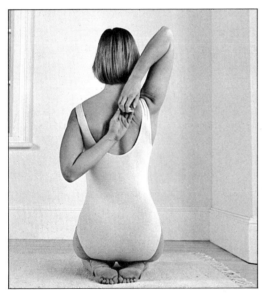

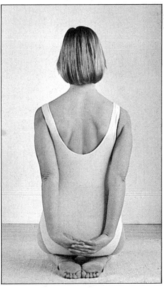

Sit on your heels on a rug, with knees together. Drop your shoulders, stretch one arm up, and bring the other up behind your back (photo at far left). On an out-breath, catch your hands, as shown on page 103. Don't drop your head forward, but extend the base of your skull toward the ceiling. Focus your attention on your breath for a few seconds. Then release your hands, and change their position. Afterward, sit quietly on your heels for a minute or two, with shoulders relaxed and eyes closed. Keep your spine straight, and clasp your hands behind you (photo at left). This will relax tight muscles in your neck. If you're still exhausted, repeat two or three times.

5 Relax

Lie on a rug on the floor, and relax as described on pages 50 and 51. Make your out-breath long and slow, easing tension in shoulders and hips. Stay in this position for 10 to 15 minutes.

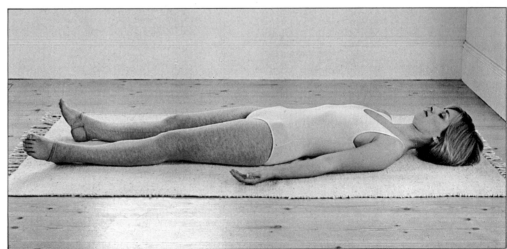

·GETTING·TO·SLEEP·

When you can't sleep your mind stays active; your body becomes more tense as you toss and turn. This program will help. Do the entire sequence just before you go to bed. If insomnia is a recurrent problem, doing a regular daily stretch program will help. See pages 58 to 73.

Caution: *Do not* stretch forward if you have a slipped disk or other acute back problem.

1 Forward and sideways

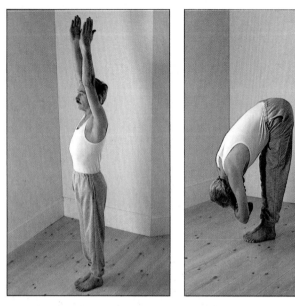

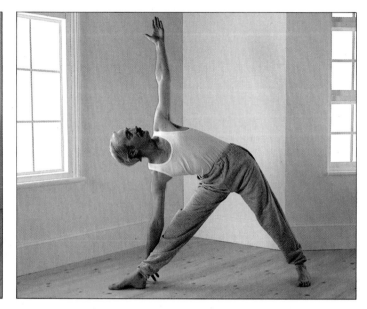

Breathe in, stand tall and stretch your arms above your head (photo above left). Breathe out, fold your arms and bend forward from your hips (photo above center). Breathe normally, stand straight, then do the basic sideways stretch as described on pages 18 and 19. Breathe out (photo above right). Hold for a few seconds, then repeat on the other side.

2 Forward and sideways

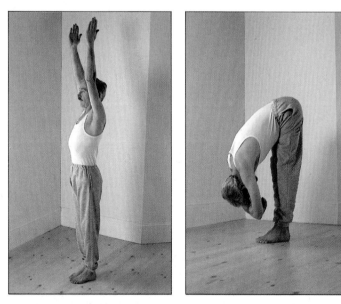

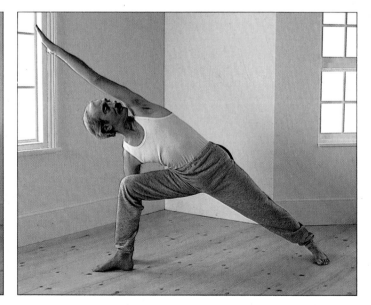

Breathe in, stand tall and stretch your arms above your head (photo at left). Breathe out, fold your arms and bend forward from your hips (photo at center). Breathe normally for a few seconds, stand straight and stretch sideways again.

Do a more advanced stretch if you can (photo at right). Breathe out as you stretch. Hold for a few seconds, then come up, and repeat on the other side.

3 Forward

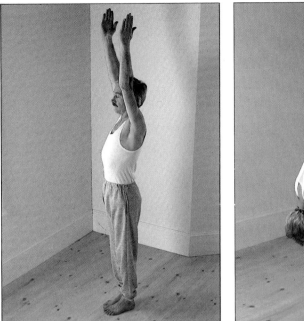

Breathe in, stand tall and stretch your arms above your head (photo above left). Breathe out, fold your arms and bend forward from your hips (photo above center). Spend at least 1 minute in this position, while breathing quietly.

4 Upside down

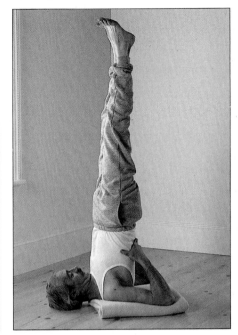

Now do the basic stretch as described on pages 42 and 43 and try to stay in this position for a few minutes. Come down slowly and carefully.

5 Relax

Sit on some pillows and stretch your trunk along your legs. Keep them straight. With each out-breath, let your body relax more completely into the position, and go to bed when you feel sleepy. Caution: If you have a back problem, use an alternative position as described on pages 52 and 53.

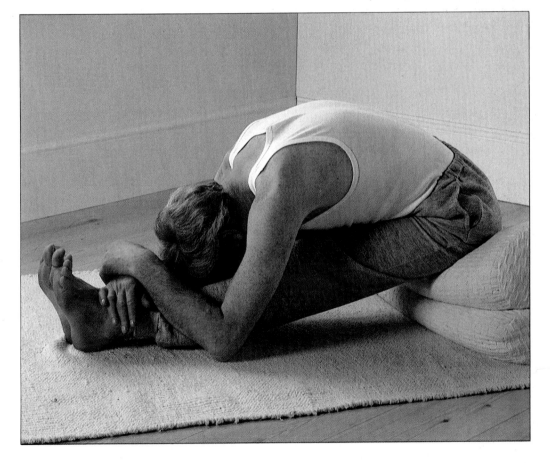

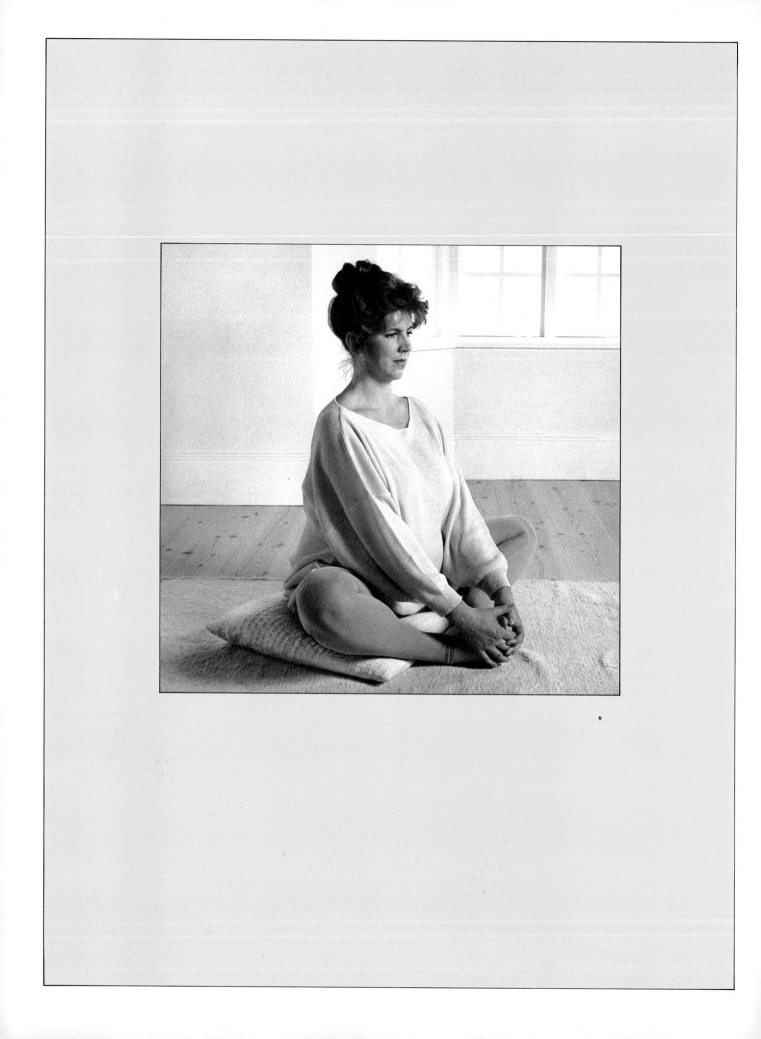

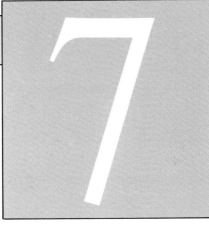

·HAVING·A·BABY·

If you're already used to practicing stretch when you become pregnant, you have a head start. You'll understand the benefits of good posture and a balanced program of exercise and relaxation. By toning your muscles and opening up your pelvic area, stretching will help prepare you for birth. It may also help relieve backache and other minor discomforts. As your baby grows larger, you should find it easy to adapt your normal daily routine, using positions for relaxation you find most comfortable.

If you're starting a stretch program in pregnancy for the first time, your increased awareness of your body will be a help. Go slowly, and thoroughly read Chapter One, so you understand the stretches before you start to practice.

During pregnancy, even women who usually find it difficult to slow down and concentrate as they stretch and relax may find a new sense of harmony with their bodies. Relaxation is essential. It brings an increased awareness of yourself and your baby. It will help you to cope with your changes of mood, and during labor, it will help you rest calmly between contractions. By practicing control over the rhythm of breathing, you'll be preparing yourself for labor. Breathing can help you feel in control of your body, even when contractions are at their strongest.

Birth is not a test to be endured and passed with top marks, and it isn't an end in itself. You may prepare yourself for a particular type of birth, then feel bitterly let down if reality is different. Try to be as open-minded as you can about labor and birth. Even if events don't match your expectations, if you exercise in pregnancy your body will be fit, well prepared and better able to cope with the demands of labor and birth. You'll probably be able to adapt stretches to the particular circumstances.

Information on pages 130 to 135 provides a stretch routine suitable for all stages of pregnancy, whether or not you have practiced stretch before. On pages 136 and 137, there is some information about positions you might find helpful in labor. On pages 138 to 143, there is a routine for the first 6 weeks after birth. After that time, you can return to a beginners' or basic stretch program. If you're in any doubt about your suitability for any of the stretches in this chapter, consult your doctor!

·STRETCH·IN·PREGNANCY·

You can probably stretch during pregnancy. You may need to include some modifications, as described in the instructions for individual stretches. Below are a few specific points to keep in mind:

1 Don't jump feet into place for standing stretches. Move smoothly into position.
2 Breathe deeply as you stretch. Make use of your breathing as you move into the positions.
3 You may find holding a position for the usual length of time is a strain. If so, do each movement briefly, but repeat it several times.
4 Stretch so you feel each stretch gives your baby more space inside you.
5 Lift up and stretch away from your pelvic floor (see below) as you move.
6 Don't lie flat on your back in late pregnancy. The baby may press against one of your major blood vessels in this position and deprive himself of oxygen or make you feel faint.

Relaxation

During the first few months of pregnancy, continue exercises to relax as usual. Use the techniques described in the chapter on relaxation (see pages 48 to 57). As the birth of your baby approaches, give more time to relaxation with deep breathing (see pages 54 to 57), prolonging only every third or fourth out-breath.

Pelvic-floor muscles

The muscles of your pelvic floor are the ones that surround the anus and vagina. You can feel them tightening if you try to stop urinating in mid-stream. During pregnancy, practice tightening and releasing these muscles several times every day called the Kegel exercise. Tighten muscles as you breathe in, and release them as you breathe out. Exercising these muscles is very important. If they become slack, sexual intercourse may become less pleasurable and, in the long-term, other problems, such as incontinence, may result. Do pelvic-floor

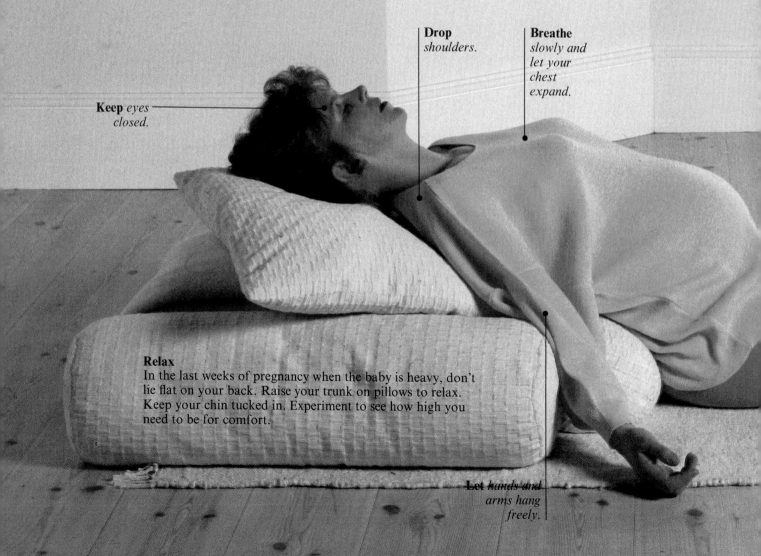

Drop *shoulders.*

Breathe *slowly and let your chest expand.*

Keep *eyes closed.*

Relax
In the last weeks of pregnancy when the baby is heavy, don't lie flat on your back. Raise your trunk on pillows to relax. Keep your chin tucked in. Experiment to see how high you need to be for comfort.

Let *hands and arms hang freely.*

exercises while doing all sorts of activities, including stretching. Begin practicing when standing straight. As you gain awareness and control of your muscles, you'll feel able to control the pelvic floor as you stretch in all directions. In labor this awareness will help you give birth with control.

Standing straight

As the baby grows, its weight pulls you forward, and the top of your spine bends back to compensate. If you stand out of alignment, the added weight of the baby puts excessive strain on the structure of your body. Instead of the spine and pelvis providing correct support, the strain will be taken by ligaments and muscles not intended for the job. If you are swaybacked, (see page 93), the curve at the back of your waist will increase, putting additional strain on the muscles of your lower back and causing backache.

Think about how you stand, not only when you're practicing stretching but in everyday life. If you are swaybacked and suffer from backache, practice the straight stretch (right) followed by relaxation (below) more than once a day.

Straight

Stand against the edge of a door, keeping your heels down. The backs of your heels, your lower back and the back of your head should touch the door. Stretch your arms up so they hold the top of the door. Loop a belt over the top if the door is too high. Breathe deeply, and enjoy stretching tall. Hold for a few seconds, then lower arms and stand as before, breathing deeply.

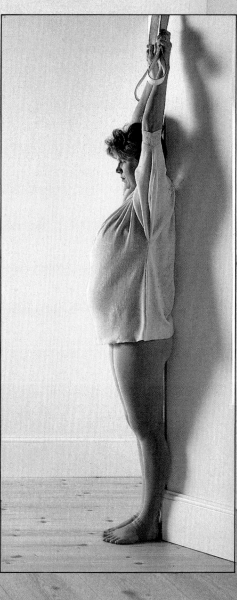

Relax *feet and toes.*

·STRETCH·IN·PREGNANCY·

The weight of the baby may pull you forward as you stretch sideways, making it hard to extend fully. Use a wall for guidance to make the correct stretch easier to feel. Don't lean on the wall. Be aware of it behind you, keeping you in line.

As you get larger, you may find the basic stretches are difficult, especially the wide-and-strong position, with hips down and knee bent. If you feel uncomfortable in any position, or if you feel you're constricting your baby, do a simple "less-stretch" movement instead of a basic stretch.

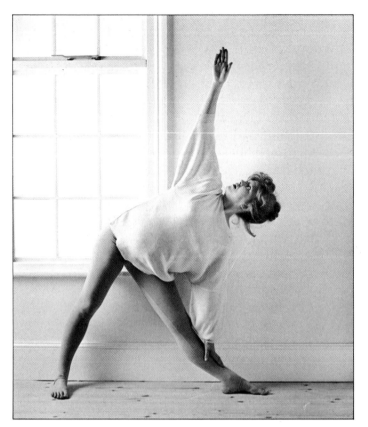

Sideways (photo at right)
Stand with a wall behind you. Follow the instructions on pages 18 and 19. The heel of your back foot should touch the wall, with your out-turned foot slightly in front of it. As you reach sideways, feel both shoulders brush the wall. Don't let yourself bend forward. Hold for a few seconds. Breathe in, come up and repeat on the other side.

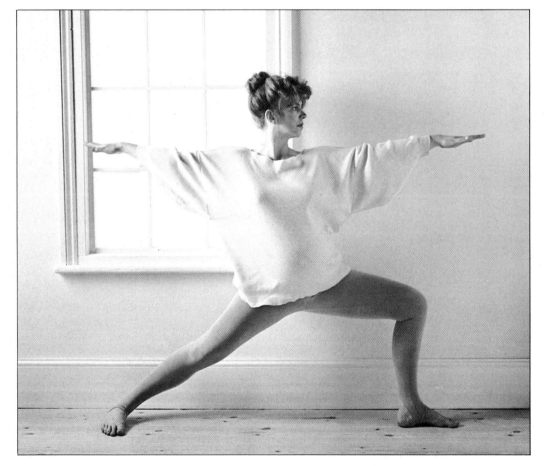

Wide and strong
With a wall behind you for guidance, follow the instructions on pages 22 and 23. Keep the heel of your back foot in contact with the wall. Place your out-turned foot a little in front of it. Lower your hips as far as you comfortably can. Lift up from your pelvic floor as you stretch up and out. Hold for a few seconds, then breathe in and come up. Repeat on the other side.

If you have practiced the basic back-to-the-center stretch regularly from the beginning of your pregnancy, balancing on one leg shouldn't be a problem, even in the last weeks. However, toward the end of pregnancy, you may prefer to stand within reach of a wall to steady yourself with one hand as you use the other to position yourself. Use the feeling of calmness you experience to focus your attention on your growing baby.

The forward stretch, shown below, is especially good for pregnancy because your arms are supported. This makes it easy to stretch and relax at the same time. With your forearms taking some of your body weight, concentrate on stretching the backs of your thighs to achieve the correct rotation of the pelvis.

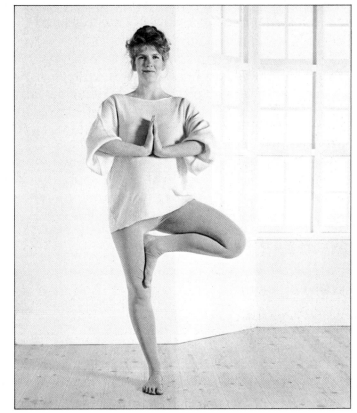

Back to the center (photo at right)
Follow the instructions on pages 26 and 27. Steady yourself against a wall with one hand if it's hard to balance on one leg. Wait until you feel secure before you align your fingers, and press your palms evenly against each other. Hold for a few seconds, breathe in and lower your foot. Repeat on the other side.

Forward
Stretch forward as far as your back-thigh muscles (hamstrings) allow you to extend. Follow the instructions on page 32. If the backs of your legs feel tight, reach out to a point high on a wall or window. If you're more supple, reach down as far as a chair seat. Lift up from your pelvic floor as you stretch. Feel the extra room for your baby as your spine extends. Hold for up to 30 seconds, then come up while breathing in.

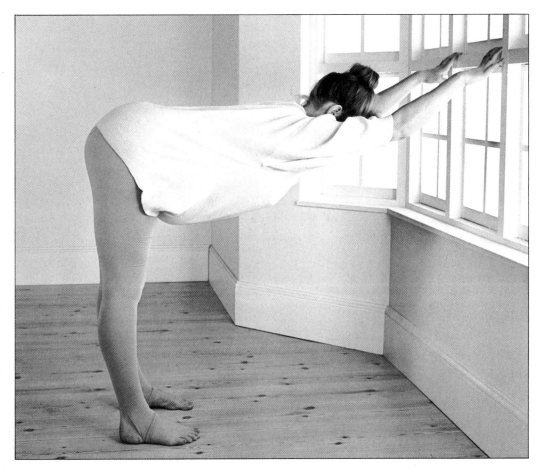

·STRETCH·IN·PREGNANCY·

There are no upside-down positions illustrated on these pages because many women find this type of stretch uncomfortable in pregnancy, and they stop doing it. This is a matter of common sense. If you wish to continue stretching upside down in pregnancy, try it after seeking professional advice. If you did not do any stretches before you became pregnant, leave upside-down positions until after birth.

Whether or not you stretch upside down after the twist and backward stretch, finish your practice with the two back-to-the-center movements shown on the opposite page. These positions loosen stiffness in the pelvis and help prepare you for the birth of your baby.

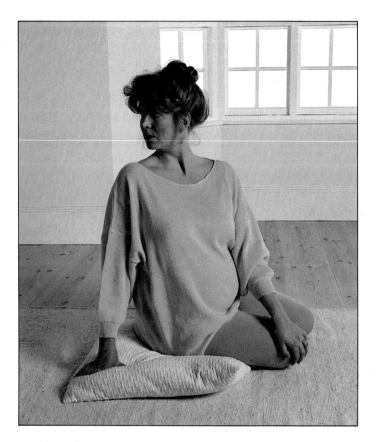

Twist (photo at right)
Sitting on a pillow, follow the instructions for the basic stretch on pages 34 and 35. Stretch up as you turn, and keep the fingertips of your right hand on the cushion or floor to help you maintain the upward lift. Hold your spine in a straight line, with the back of your head directly above the back of your hips. Stay in the position for a few seconds. Breathe in and come up. Repeat on the other side.

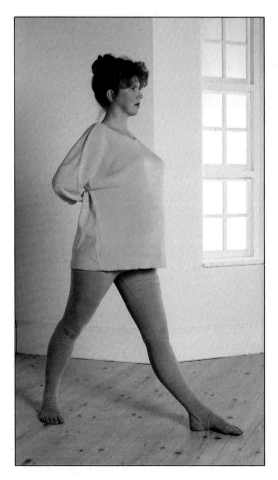

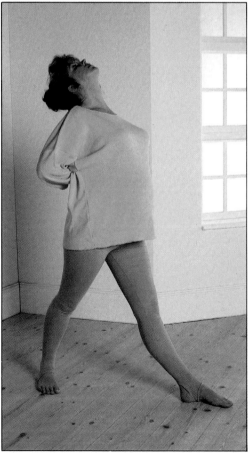

Backward
Spread your feet 36 inches apart. Turn your right foot slightly in and your left heel with your right arch. Turn your trunk to the left. Rest your arms behind you, and turn your hands up, fingers pointing up and palms together. Press your palms against each other, and move your elbows back (photo at far left).

Stretch up, breathing in. Then breathe out, and bend back. Your lower spine should extend as you stretch up. Your upper back should lift and stretch backward as you continue to press your hands together (photo at left). Hold for a few seconds, breathe in and come back to a vertical position. Take two or three deep breaths, and repeat on the other side.

Note: If you're unable to put your hands up behind your back, hold your elbows behind your waist instead.

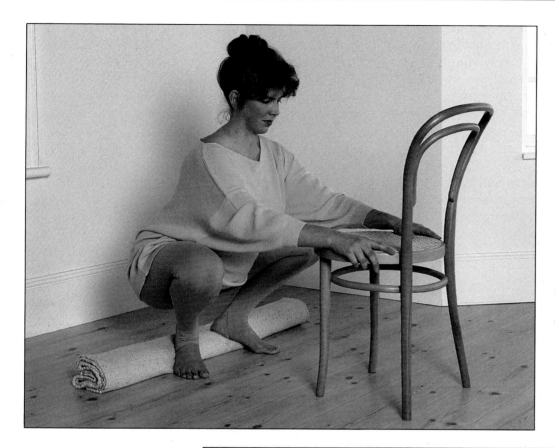

Back to the center
Stand facing a chair with your feet about 12 inches apart. Bend at your hips and knees. Squat down, holding the chair to steady yourself. Try to keep feet flat on the floor; if this is impossible, put a folded blanket under your heels. Press your heels down, and open out your knees, keeping your back straight. Breathe quietly, and hold for as long as you comfortably can. When you can stay in this position for 30 seconds and keep your balance, do it without the chair. This is a good position for practicing pelvic-floor exercises – see page 130.

Back to the center
Follow the instructions on page 29. Put a pillow under your buttocks if hip joints are not flexible or if your lower back tends to collapse. Do the stretch more than once a day if you can. Hold it for a few seconds longer each time you practice.

Although this position may be difficult, you may find it easier than you imagine because pelvic joints become more flexible in pregnancy.

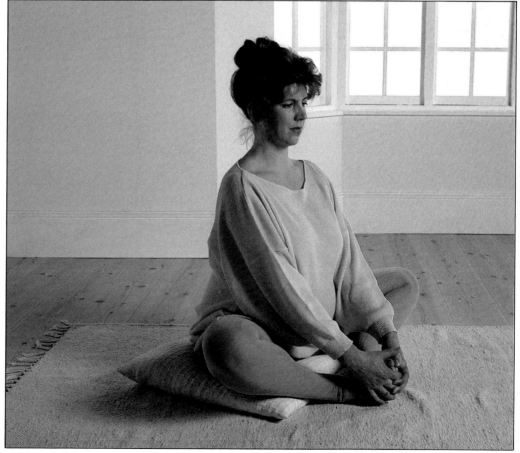

·POSITIONS·FOR·LABOR·

Stretching and relaxing during pregnancy will extend into preparation for labor. By the time your baby is born, you should have an understanding of your body, and know how to relax and tune in to your breathing.

Animals instinctively find the most comfortable, convenient way to deliver their young, and women need to be free to do the same during labor. Over the years, various considerations – including fashion and the convenience of medical attendants – have dictated the positions and movements of mothers during childbirth. By restricting women to unsuitable positions, certain techniques have even added to the distress they were intended to alleviate.

However, it has been suggested recently that allowing and encouraging women to be active in labor has not only made deliveries quicker and less painful, but it has reduced the need for medical intervention.

Labor is a time to feel free and uninhibited. Because social custom usually restricts you to certain forms of behavior, you may not be used to spontaneity in your movements. It's a good idea, during pregnancy, to practice various positions you might find helpful in labor and to imagine how you might want to behave during intense contractions. You may find some illustrated positions relaxing when you want to rest in the last few weeks; it can be hard to get comfortable when your baby is large.

The best positions in labor are those in which the pull of gravity assists the delivery of the baby. Sitting back on your tailbone, for instance, is *not* a good position because your tailbone impedes the passage of the baby. Lying flat on your back is not good either because you must push against gravity, and the baby may become short of oxygen. In the first stage, move around as much as you are able to. Adopt many different positions. As birth draws closer, and you find it harder to move around, try to settle in a position where your pelvis is free to open naturally.

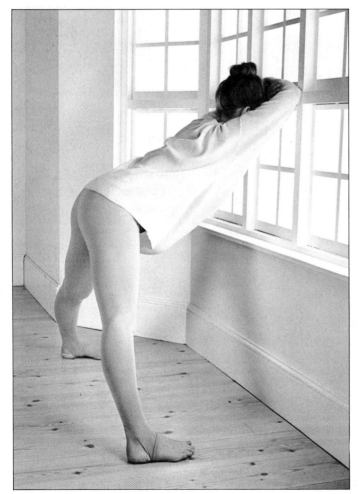

Forward (photo at left)
Try stretching up and forward, with feet apart. Rest comfortably against a wall or a window, and cradle your head in your arms. If you prefer, stretch your arms out.

Sitting (photo below)
Sit on a straight-backed chair. Rest your head on your arms supported by pillows, with your feet flat on the floor. Put a cushion on the chair seat if you want to.

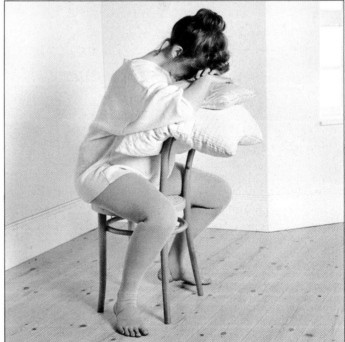

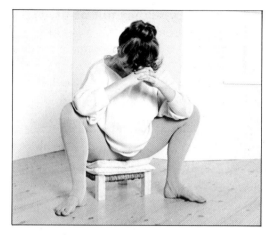

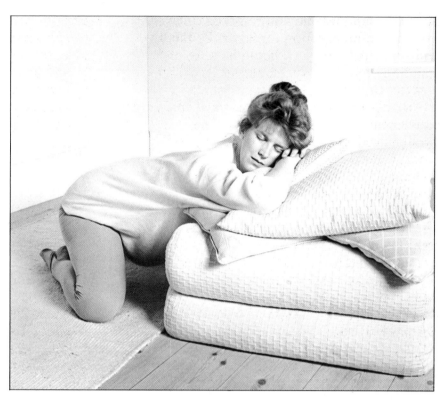

Squatting (photo above)
Lower yourself into a squatting position. Place some pillows on a low stool under your buttocks for support. With your feet flat on the floor, rest your elbows on your knees and your head on your hands.

Kneeling onto pillows (photo at right)
Kneel with your knees wide apart. Rest your head and arms on a pile of pillows.

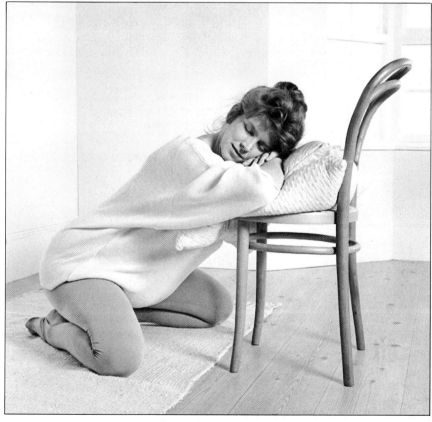

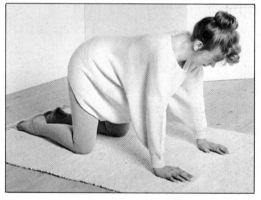

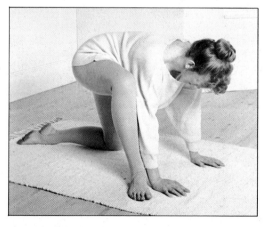

Kneeling onto a chair
Spread your knees wide apart. Kneel with your head and arms resting on a chair seat. Use pillows for support. Keeping your body vertical can help speed up labor.

On all fours
Kneel on all fours. Let your spine extend by rocking, if this is helpful (photo at top). You may prefer one knee bent (photo above).

·AFTER·BIRTH·

Most new mothers are unprepared for the tiredness of the first few days – and often weeks – after birth. Giving birth takes all your physical and emotional strength. You and your baby need time to adapt to life as two separate people. For a few weeks, try to avoid too many outside pressures; adjust to your new rhythm at your own pace.

With a small baby, your daily routine will be different. You may find it difficult to stretch and relax, especially if you have other children. But stretch will repay you for your time with energy and strength. If you were very fit and active before the birth, practicing stretch regularly, the post-natal exercises will be easier. You'll quickly regain your shape and fitness, as day by day you retone your muscles.

Deliveries vary, so how soon you can do a particular stretch depends on you. If some of the stretches don't feel right, do simpler movements for a few days. Repeat them often. Use your common sense, and introduce new movements when you feel ready. If you had a Cesarean delivery, you *must* consult your obstetrician before you begin any exercises.

The following pages suggest a program of exercises for the first 6 weeks or so after you have your baby. Each week introduces some new movements into a suggested daily routine, and these new movements are picked out by a colored border. When instructions to the stretches refer to a basic stretch from Chapter One, substitute a "less-stretch" movement if this is more suited to your usual stretch level. At the end of 6 weeks, start a complete beginners' or basic program. Continue to include shoulder stretches and pelvic-floor exercises. If you were doing a more advanced program before you became pregnant, you can return to it 3 months after birth.

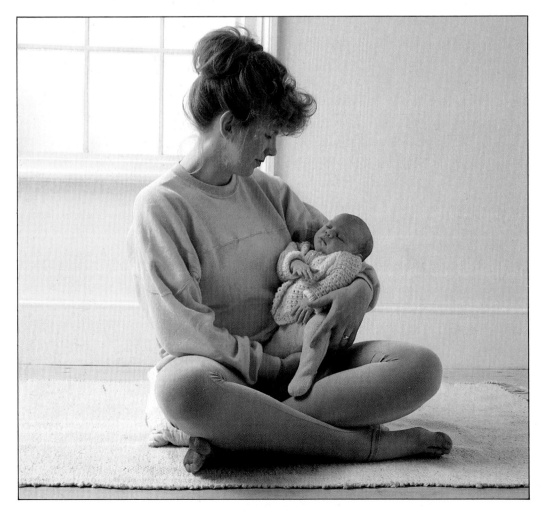

Mother and child
The time you give to stretching and relaxation can reward you with renewed energy. You'll enjoy your new baby in the very first weeks of his or her life.

·WEEK·ONE·

1 Straight

Lie on your back on a rug, with knees bent and arms stretched above your head (photo above right). Keep the back of your waist flat on the floor. Slowly straighten your legs, keeping your waist extended (photo below right). Tighten your abdominal muscles and your pelvic-floor muscles. See page 130. Stretch from your heels to your fingertips for a few seconds. Relax, and repeat several times.

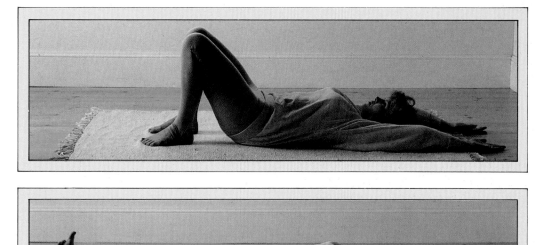

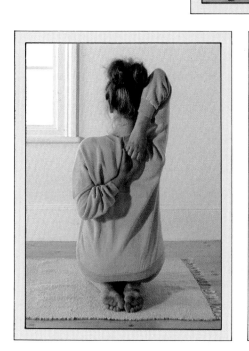 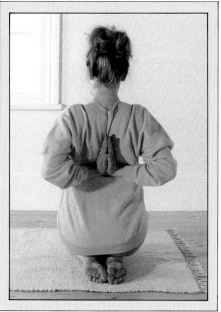

2 Shoulders

Sit on your heels, and clasp your hands behind your back (see photo at far left), as described on page 103. Hold for a few seconds, then repeat with hands the other way around. Next, fold your hands behind your back with palms together (photo at left). As you stretch your elbows back, breathe deeply and open your chest. Hold for a few seconds, relax, then repeat once or twice.

These shoulder stretches are important if you breast-feed your baby and bend over a lot.

3 Relax

Lie on your back on the floor to relax. If this is uncomfortable, choose an alternate position from pages 52 and 53. Stay in the positions for 5 to 10 minutes.

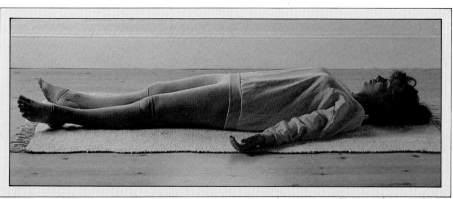

·WEEK·TWO·

1 Straight

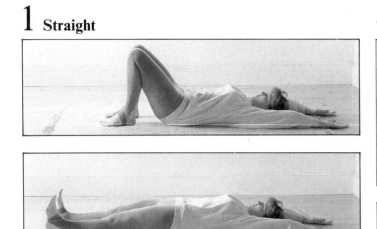

2 Shoulders

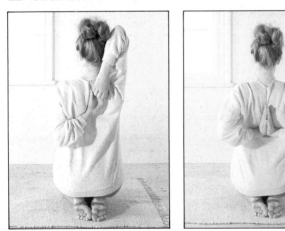

3 Forward

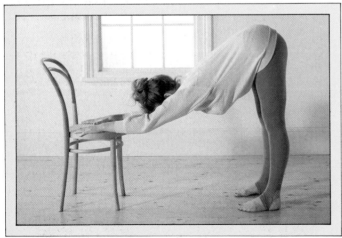

Bend forward from your hips, as shown on page 32. Breathe deeply. At the end of an out-breath, pull your abdominal muscles in strongly toward your spine. At the same time, squeeze your pelvic-floor muscles. Relax your grip as you breathe in. Take a few deep breaths. Repeat and come up.

4 Backward

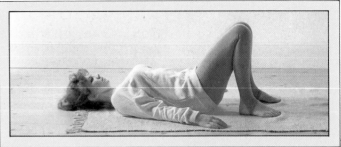

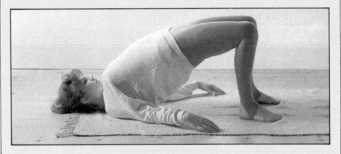

Lie on your back on a rug with your knees bent (photo at top). Take a few deep breaths, then lift your hips on an out-breath. Tuck in your tailbone, and tighten your buttock muscles (photo above). Keep your arms on the floor. Hold for a few seconds, then breathe in and come down.

5 Back to the center

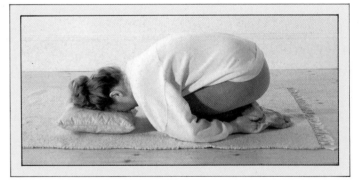

Kneel and bend forward, as shown on page 28. Keep your buttocks down on your heels, and relax your neck and shoulders. Hold for a few seconds, breathe in and come up.

6 Relax

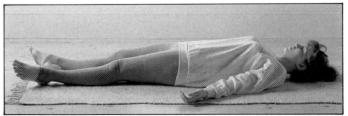

· WEEK · THREE ·

1 Straight

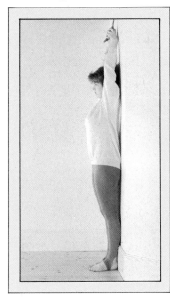

Stand up, and stretch tall (photo at left). Use the edge of the door as you did when you were pregnant. See page 131. Tighten your pelvic-floor muscles and abdominal muscles in the same way as you did when lying flat.

Stand straight to do shoulder stretches from Weeks 1 and 2 (photos at right and far right). Hold each stretch for a few seconds; repeat several times.

2 Shoulders

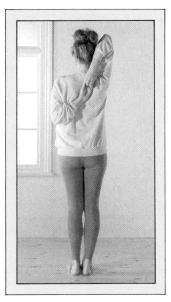
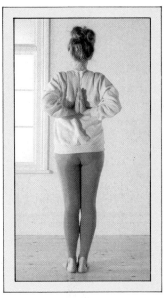

3 Forward

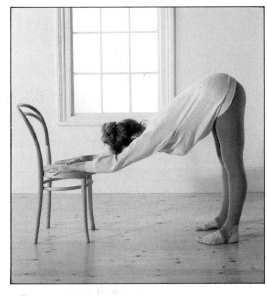

4 Twist

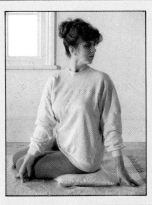

Do the basic twist, as described on pages 34 and 35. Hold for a few seconds, then breathe in and face forward again.

5 Backward

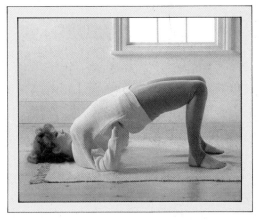

Do the stretch you started in Week 2. If you lift your hips high enough, support your back with your hands. Hold for a few seconds, then breathe in and come down.

6 Back to the center

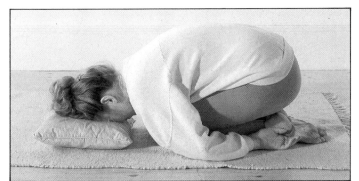

7 Relax

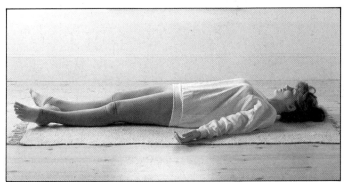

·WEEK·FOUR·

1 Straight
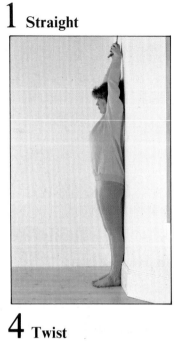

2 Shoulders
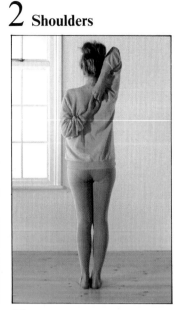

3 Forward
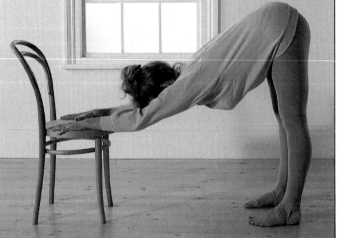

4 Twist
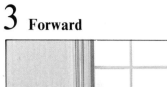

5 Backward
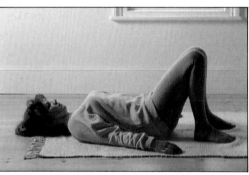
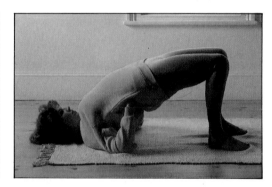

6 Backward
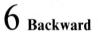
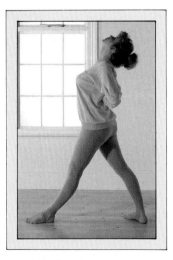

7 Back to the center
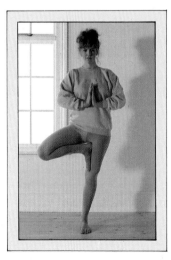

8 Back to the center
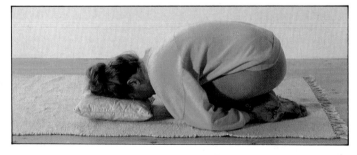

9 Relax
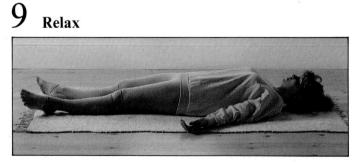

Add the stretch you did when pregnant. See page 134. Hold for a few seconds, then breathe in and come up.

Do the basic stretch on pages 26 and 27. Hold for a few seconds, then repeat, standing on the other leg.

·WEEKS·FIVE & SIX·

1 Straight

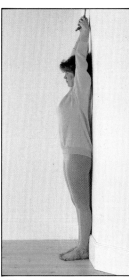

2 Shoulders

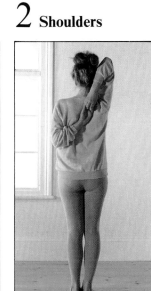

3 Sideways

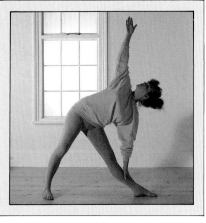

Add the basic stretch on pages 18 and 19. Hold for a few seconds. Breathe in, come up and repeat on the other side.

4 Back to the center

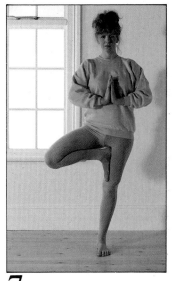

5 Forward

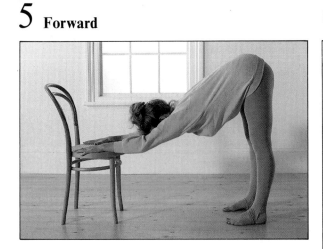

6 Twist

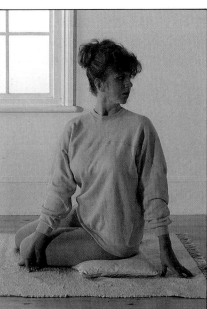

7 Backward

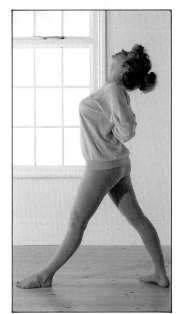

8 Upside down

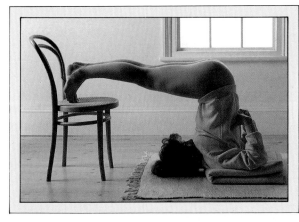

Include the basic position from pages 42 and 43. Hold for a few minutes. Then place your feet back on a chair (see page 46) for a few seconds. Bend your knees over your head, and roll gently down.

9 Relax

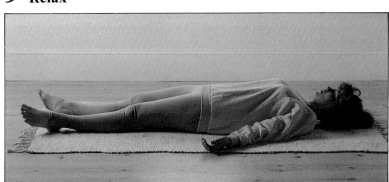

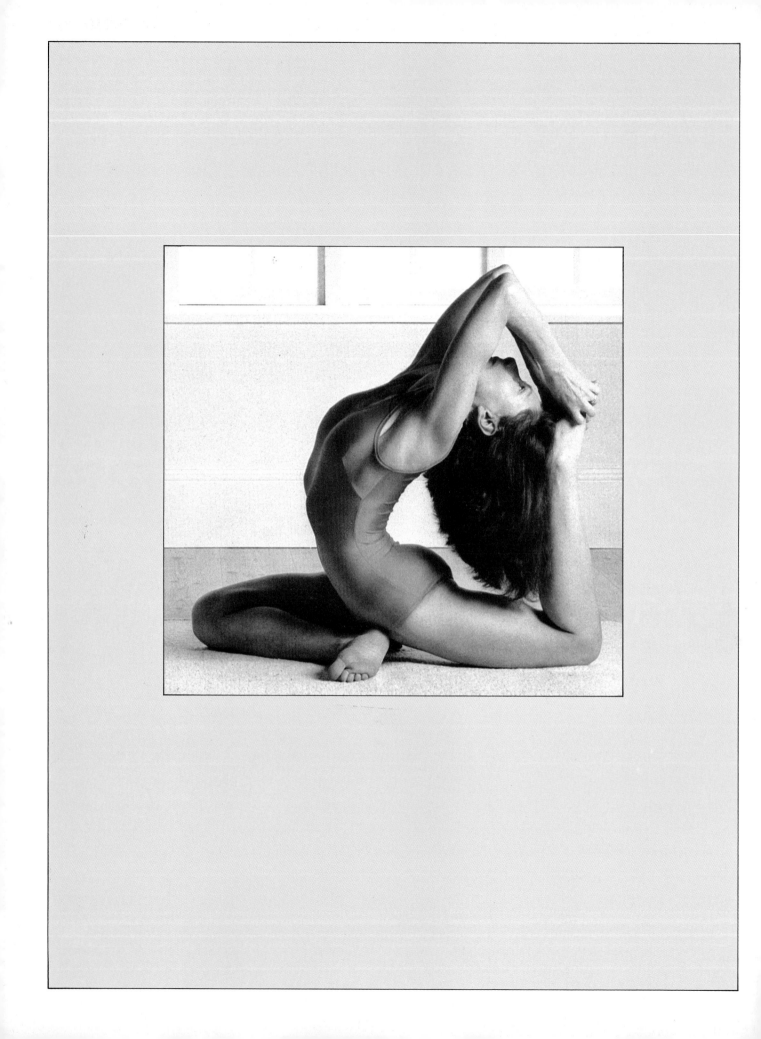

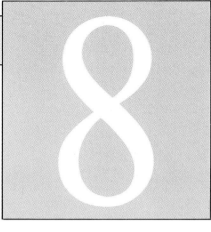

· STRETCH · MORE ·

The intense stretches described in this chapter are for people who enjoy the freedom of movement that stretching brings, who can do all the other stretches in this book with ease and who would like to stretch more. Although it's possible to practice by yourself, it is safer to have some expert guidance. If you want to embark on an advanced stretching program, the help of an experienced teacher is invaluable.

The stretches in this chapter are not suitable for inclusion in a 20-minute daily program. To extend the body this far with safety, you need to warm up gradually and take time to relax fully afterward. A sudden stretch when the body is unprepared can cause injury. It's impossible to give a warm-up routine to suit everyone because flexibility differs from person to person. Everybody needs to warm up in different ways. Working with a good teacher will help you evolve a warm-up routine and practice to suit your own particular body type.

Advanced stretches must be part of a regular daily discipline; this takes a lot of time and dedication. It isn't safe to do them occasionally, when you have a little more time to spare. If you stretch in an intense practice only once a week, the following day your body would feel bruised and exhausted instead of free and relaxed. It isn't sensible to practice the stretches individually, however easy you may find a specific movement. Daily practice is essential, because stretching in this chapter is the culmination of continuous regular practice of the other stretches in this book. These advanced stretches should be part of a weekly routine where daily programs are adapted, so a different stretch can be practiced each day.

All the stretches in this chapter must be preceded by less intense movements of the same type and followed by counter-movements, upside-down stretches and a long period of relaxation. To understand the movements of your own body and the correct action of the stretches, you need a great deal of time and patience and the help of a teacher. Although these are difficult and demanding stretches, expert help, time and dedication can bring them within the range of many more people than is generally realized.

·SIDEWAYS·

The first stretch involves an intense sideways stretch in the spine. Hips remain straight while your spine extends. In the second position, you stretch your whole body sideways. If you keep your shoulders back correctly, as in the basic sideways stretch, this movement should be easy.

First stretch

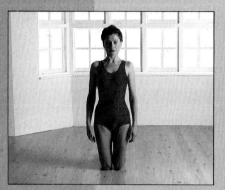

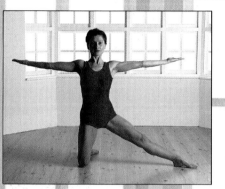

1 Kneel with your tailbone tucked in and the tops of your feet flat on the floor behind you. Stretch up through your spine.

2 Extend your left leg. Keep the heel of your left foot in line with your right knee. Drop your shoulders, and stretch your arms out, palms up.

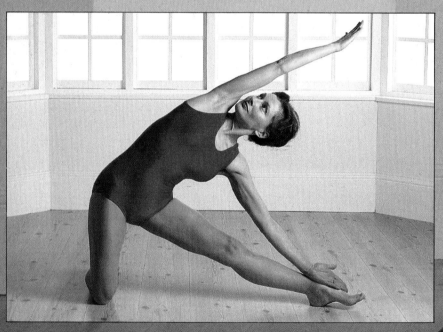

3 Breathing out, extend your trunk to the left. Stretch from your hips until the back of your left hand rests on your left foot. Keeping your right thigh vertical, stretch from your lower back. Bring your right arm over your head. Extend through the fingertips of that arm, feeling the stretch in the ribcage as you do this. Breathe normally for a few seconds, then come up while breathing in. Repeat on the other side.

Second stretch

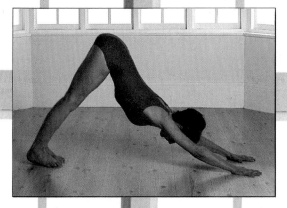

1 Lie on your front on the floor with your hands under your chest, fingers pointing forward. On an out-breath, lift your hips so your trunk and legs make a triangle with the floor. Keep your heels on the floor.

Keep *upper arm in line with lower arm.*

2 Keeping your left arm strong, raise your right hand. Turn your entire body to the right, while keeping your feet together. Your hips and shoulders should be in line. Turn your head to look up at your right hand. Hold for a few seconds. Then come up while breathing in. Repeat on the other side.

Lift *hips.*

Feel *chest open.*

Extend *back of head.*

Stretch *knees and keep legs straight.*

·WIDE & STRONG·

This position involves an intense stretch in the
thigh muscles and requires strong back muscles.
The full split position should be attempted *only* by
experienced students under the guidance of a
teacher. Practice slowly, and never force yourself.

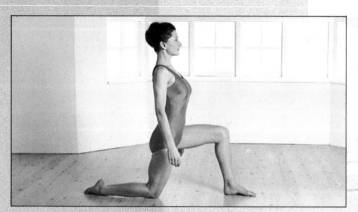

1 Kneel on one knee. Face
forward, keeping your
hips straight. Stretch up
through your spine. Open
your chest as you breathe in.

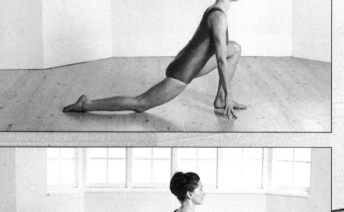

2 On an out-breath, bend
forward, and put your
hands on the floor. Keep
your spine stretched from
tailbone to head. Don't
tighten neck or shoulders.

3 Breathe in. As you
breathe out again, slide
your front leg forward.
Support your weight with
your hands. Keep your hips
facing forward as far as
possible and let your back
leg straighten. Your back
knee should face the floor,
your front knee the ceiling.

Keep *back
knee facing
floor.*

Use *stretch of arms to pull up spine.*

4 Let your hips settle on the floor, and take a few breaths. Breathe in, and feel your spine stretch up. On an out-breath, raise your arms above your head, with palms together. Keep the lift in the back of your body. Hold for a few seconds before releasing, then come up. Repeat with the other leg in front.

Lift *back ribs.*

Stretch *up from floor through spine.*

Extend *heel of front leg.*

Rotate *back hip forward.*

·BACK·TO·THE·CENTER·

This stretch is a continuation of the "more-stretch" position described on page 29. You need a flexible back and hips to do it. If you get a cramp as a result of bending your spine instead of stretching it, come up and lie flat with knees bent.

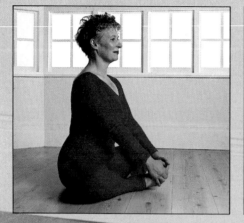

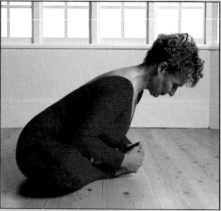

1 Sit with your knees bent, feet together, close to your body, and your back straight. Keep your shoulders relaxed, and let both thighs drop down toward the floor.

2 Holding your feet, breathe out and stretch forward. Extend the entire front of your trunk. Continue to drop your thighs toward the floor.

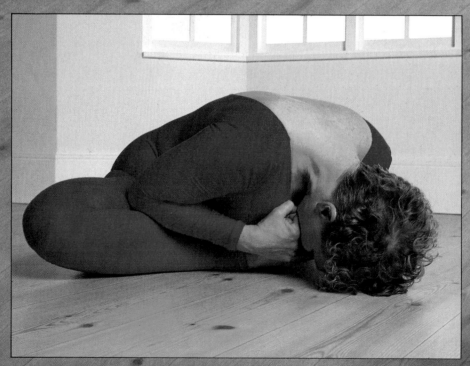

3 Rest your head on the floor. Your entire spine should be stretched and your chest open. Hold the position for two or three breaths, then breathe in and come up.

·FORWARD·

This stretch takes a lot of time and patience because the insides of your thighs and knees need to extend. Never force or strain to do this stretch. Allow your legs to stretch gradually in the basic and "more-stretch" positions (see pages 30 to 33).

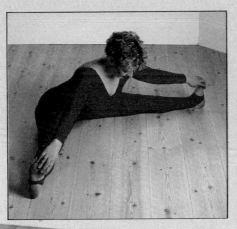

1 Sit with your legs wide apart, so you face the center between your feet. Extend your heels, and straighten your knees. Catch your feet with your hands. Feel your lower back move up and in before you go any farther.

2 Put your hands in front of you on the floor. Keep the front of your body extended, and stretch forward. Your spine should lengthen as you breathe in.

Keep *buttock bones pressing against floor.*

Extend *entire spine.*

Stretch *heels strongly.*

Relax *back of neck.*

Stretch *arms wide and open chest.*

3 As you breathe out, go farther forward, and reach your hands to your feet. Don't pull forward with your hands, but stretch from your lower spine. On the next out-breath, put your head and chest on the floor. Hold for a second or two, breathe in and come up.

·TWIST·

This standing twist demands flexible hips so as your upper back turns, your chest stays open and unconstricted. Turn from your hips without forcing or pushing your shoulders hard against the outside of your knee. At first you'll take several breaths as you move into the stretch, but eventually you'll be able to do the entire movement in one breath.

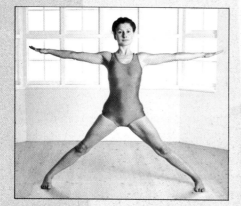

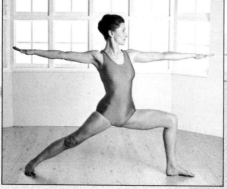

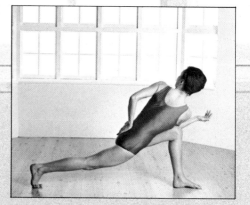

1 Stand tall and straight. Stretch up through the curves of your spine. Spread your feet wide apart, and keep the stretch in your back. Extend your arms at shoulder level, and stretch into your fingertips. Keep the palms of your hands facing the floor.

2 Turn your right foot slightly in and your left leg out. Align your left heel with the arch of your right foot. Turn your head to the left, as you bend your left knee and lower your hips. Keep the stretch wide and strong.

3 Lift your right heel; on an out-breath turn your trunk to the left. Keep your left thigh parallel to the floor and your knee back. Place your left hand on your hip, then reach behind your left knee with your right arm.

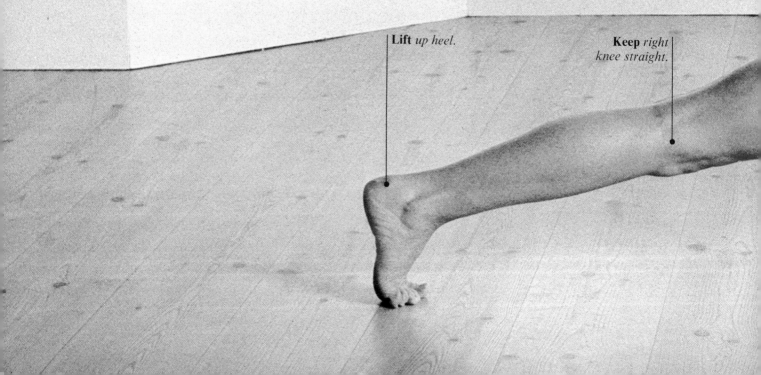

Lift *up heel.*

Keep *right knee straight.*

Stretch *upper arm into fingertips.*

Make sure *left hip stays down.*

Feel *ribs move over left thigh.*

4 Straighten your right arm so fingers rest on the floor. The outside of your left knee should touch the back of your right shoulder. Keep your right leg straight and stretched toward the heel. On the next out-breath, take your left shoulder back. Stretch your left arm over your head, with palm down. You'll feel the stretch along your entire body from right heel to left hand.

·BACKWARD·

In these advanced stretches, it's essential for your entire spine to stretch as you extend backward. You need flexible hips, shoulders and a flexible upper back to do this exercise, or you'll feel constricted at the waist.

First stretch

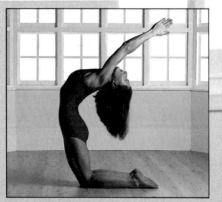

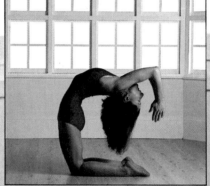

1 Kneel and stretch up, as if preparing to do the basic stretch on page 38. Tilt your head back, and lift away from your hips. Curve your upper back, and open your chest.

2 Let your arms bend as you continue to extend backward. Keep your hips forward, with your weight on your knees and feet. Stretch slowly, with control.

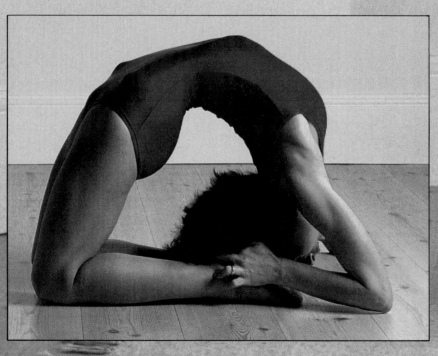

3 Hold your feet with your hands. Open your chest, and move hips forward. Curve your spine so your head rests on your feet with your elbows on the floor. Hold for a few seconds, then come up while breathing in.

Second stretch

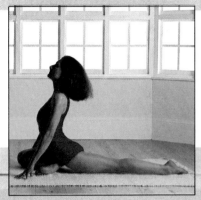 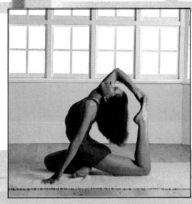

1 Lie on your front on a rug. Fold right leg in front of you, and extend your left leg. Place your hands on the floor, and lift your trunk. Keep your hips straight so your lower back is evenly stretched.

2 Bend your left leg. Breathing in, stretch your spine up and back. Stretch your right arm over your head. On an out-breath, catch your left foot.

3 Keeping your left leg strong, take your left arm over your head and grasp your foot. Breathing out, curve your upper back, and extend your neck. Move your head back until your foot touches the top of your head. Hold for a few seconds, then let go of the foot one hand at a time. Breathe in, and bring your head slowly up.

Stretch *back foot.*

Make sure *right hip stays back.*

Feel *left hip come forward.*

Keep *top of knee flat on floor.*

·INDEX·

·ACKNOWLEDGMENTS·

Dorling Kindersley would like to thank the following for their special assistance: Jeff Veitch for the photography; Kris Watson for constructing the set; Adrian Ensor for the black and white prints; Karen Cochrane for the illustrations; Ken Hone for retouching; Chambers Wallace for typesetting; Richard and Hilary Bird for the index; Armstrong Flooring; Beverly of "Splitz"; Dr Cathy Bond; Alison Chappel; Christine Coleman; Dr Keith Fairweather; Fenwicks; Hilary Guy; Dr Faith Haddad; Nathalie of Joan Price's "The Face Place"; Pineapple; Dianne Scrivener.

·MARY·STEWART·   ·MAXINE·TOBIAS·

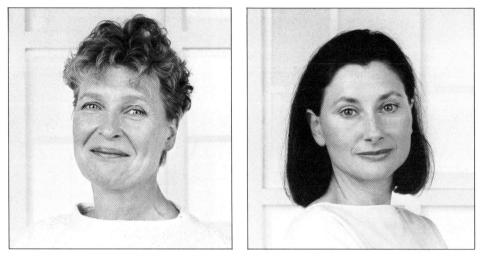

Health, Sports and Fitness Books from The Body Press

Complete Guide to Prescription & Non-Prescription Drugs – Griffith **$12.95**
High-Performance Racquetball – Hogan **$8.95**
Low-Stress Fitness – Brown **$8.95**
MuscleAerobics – Patano & Savage **$8.95**
Stretch & Relax – Tobias & Stewart **$12.95**
Symptoms, Illness & Surgery – Griffith **$12.95**
Pregnant & Beautiful – Curtis, Hazeltine, Rasband **$8.95**

The Body Press books are available wherever fine books are sold, or order direct from the publisher. Send check or money order payable in U.S. funds to: The Body Press, P.O. Box 5367, Dept. STR-A5, Tucson, AZ 85703 Include $1.95 postage and handling for first book; $1.00 for each additional book. Arizona residents add 7% sales tax. Please allow 4-6 weeks for delivery. Prices subject to change without notice.

·CONVERSION TO METRIC MEASURE·

When You Know	Symbol	Multiply By	To Find	Symbol
VOLUME				
teaspoons	tsp.	4.93	milliliters	ml
tablespoons	tbsp.	14.79	milliliters	ml
fluid ounces	fl. oz.	29.57	milliliters	ml
cups	c.	0.24	liters	l
pints	pt.	0.47	liters	l
quarts	qt.	0.95	liters	l
gallons	gal.	3.79	liters	l
LENGTH				
inches	in.	2.54	centimeters	cm
feet	ft.	30.48	centimeters	cm
yards	yd.	0.91	meters	m
TEMPERATURE				
Fahrenheit	F	0.56 (after subtracting 32)	Celsius	C